Beautiful Brain, Beautiful You

Look Radiant from
the Inside Out by
Empowering Your Mind

Marie Pasinski, M.D.

WITH JODIE GOULD

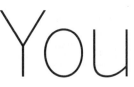

voice

Hyperion • New York

Copyright © 2011 Harvard University

All rights reserved. No part of this book may be used or reproduced in any manner whatsoever without the written permission of the Publisher. Printed in the United States of America. For information address Hyperion, 114 Fifth Avenue, New York, New York, 10011.

Library of Congress Cataloging-in-Publication Data

Pasinski, Marie.
  Beautiful brain, beautiful you : look radiant from the inside out by empowering your mind / Marie Pasinski with Jodie Gould.
      p. cm.
  Includes bibliographical references.
  ISBN 978-1-4013-4148-0
  1. Brain. 2. Women—Health and hygiene. 3. Beauty, Personal. 4. Neuroplasticity. I. Gould, Jodie. II. Title.
  QP376.P366 2011
  612.8'2—dc22

                                                  2010035209

Hyperion books are available for special promotions and premiums. For details contact the HarperCollins Special Markets Department in the New York office at 212-207-7528, fax 212-207-7222, or email spsales@harpercollins.com.

                    FIRST EDITION

          10 9 8 7 6 5 4 3 2 1

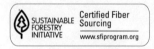

THIS LABEL APPLIES TO TEXT STOCK

To the men in my life,
my husband, Roger,
and my sons, Eric and Stephen,
with gratitude and love.

And to all women everywhere,
may you nurture and celebrate the
true beauty of your brain.

—MP

To my beloved family (brainiacs all),
and to all the brilliant and radiant women.
May your mind, body, and spirit
stay forever young.

—JG

CONTENTS

Beautiful Brain, Beautiful You

The Beauty/Brain Connection

Beauty is how you feel inside, and it reflects in your eyes.
It is not something physical.
—SOPHIA LOREN, ACTRESS

In the search for that magic lotion or potion that will make us more beautiful, I'm here to tell you that the answer lies inside your head. That's right—your brain is the key to improving every facet of your life. It generates your thoughts, emotions, actions, reactions, moods, dreams, and creative ideas. It holds all the memories, experiences, and knowledge that you have accumulated since you were born. It interprets every sensation you experience and controls each movement you make. It allows you to learn and to remember, and it ultimately determines whether you will live a productive and meaningful life. Your brain is your essence, and it is also the essence of your beauty. By enhancing your mind you can feel more energetic, creative, and alive—all of which makes you more beautiful!

In my training at Harvard Medical School and neurology practice at Massachusetts General Hospital, I have been fortunate to witness and contemplate the beauty of the human brain. I wrote this book so I could share the empowering knowledge of what you can do to get your brain in peak condition and keep it that way for life. Other brain books will advise you to challenge your brain with puzzles and memory games. While these might be helpful, I encourage you to embark

1

on a wider journey that includes optimizing the lifestyle and health factors that impact your brain function, as well as pursuing adventure and enriching yourself by trying new activities that will challenge and expand your mind.

Beautiful Brain, Beautiful You is a guide to achieving your personal best brain. By following my seven-step program, you will learn how to reap the benefits of a healthy, active, vibrant mind at any age. With your brain at its best, your ability to think creatively, make wise decisions, and problem solve will improve. Your mind will be focused, your mood high, and your self-confidence boosted. What could be more attractive?

So how can we tap into the beauty/brain connection? It starts with understanding how your face mirrors the chemical activity going on in your brain. This activity produces microfacial expressions—the tiny involuntary reflections of your thoughts that radiate from within and give you that inner glow, which we will talk more about later. By transforming the workings of your inner mind and altering the way you think, you can change the way you present yourself to the world.

Consider how you look after you've stayed up too late or had a few too many glasses of wine. Chances are you are not at your best. When your thoughts are sluggish and your mood is low, the twinkle in your eye that you have when you are at the top of your game disappears. This is what I call a "Bad Brain Day." We all have them. Whether we call it Mommy Brain, PMS, or Senior Moments, these are the times when we are running on empty and our brain finds it harder to muster the energy to get through the day. Fortunately there are concrete steps you can take to improve your brain performance, uplift your mood, and trigger creative thinking.

The beauty of the brain is that the more you use it, the stronger and more resilient it will become. Unlike a road that becomes riddled with potholes the more it's used, neural pathways actually get reinforced and become more flexible with use. The scientific term for this is neuroplasticity—the brain's ability to remodel itself by making new connections as well as new neurons. We once believed that we were born with all the brain cells we would ever have in our lifetime. We now know that our brain is a fertile field that is capable of producing new cells and creating new connections throughout our lives. What makes this such an exciting new discovery is that we now know it's possible to keep our brain vibrant and supple as we get older.

When we put on makeup, we are creating a superficial kind of beauty that is erased as soon as it is washed off. But when you give your brain that much-needed makeover, the changes that occur are profound and everlasting. Your brain is constantly evolving below the surface so that your inner beauty can shine through. By providing a luxuriant, nurturing environment, your mind will thrive and remain youthful.

A beauty/brain makeover involves "indulging in the new," because the more you learn, the easier it is to learn more. In this book, you will discover what happens to your brain when you are exposed to something new, and why your brain is the gift that keeps on giving. I will explain how physical ailments, mood disorders, hormones, and medications directly affect brain performance. I will also tell you which supplements work and which do not, and how the beauty we see on the outside is a direct reflection of what's happening on the inside.

Ever wonder why it's so hard to lose those extra ten pounds? It has to do with your brain! I will show you how changing the way you think can help you change your brain and your body. I will ask you to take better care of your health by getting your heart pumping, which improves blood flow to your brain and encourages the growth of new neurons and new brain pathways. I will explain why having the proper mind-set will help you to lose that unhealthy weight you might be carrying around. By controlling your mind, you can change your negative behavior, thoughts, and actions. The same goes for adopting the the Smart Diet, which will help boost your brain function while trimming your waistline.

You will also discover how to "make over your mind" by engaging in relaxation techniques that relieve stress, improve mood, and enhance mental clarity. Similarly, you will have a new understanding of how to beautify your brain rhythms through restorative sleep and how to synchronize your brain's internal clocks, which influence your concentration, energy, hunger, libido, and emotions.

While reading this, I hope you will be inspired to make the most of your brain—our most precious gift. Once you notice the change in the way you feel and the way you look (and others start noticing as well!), I hope that you will help spread the word to other women about how gorgeous their minds can be, and how the lifestyle choices they make can transform their brain and appearance from dull to dazzling. As much fun as a brain makeover can be, there is no quick fix for a Bad Brain Day. Some of the lifestyle changes in my program will require more time and effort on your part. Still, as you progress in the program, you will start replacing Bad Brain Days with Beautiful Brain Days by tapping into your brain's ability to change and renew itself. By the end of the book, you will discover the richness of your mind's unlimited potential and realize that you can achieve your personal best only when your brain is at its personal best. When this happens, you will see why the most powerful kind of beauty is the one that emanates from within.

Picture Perfect
(A Beauty/Brain Exercise)

Look at several photographs of yourself at different stages in your life. Now select the ones where you appear the most radiant—ones in which you have that special gleam in your eye. What's happening in the photo? What were you thinking when the shutter clicked? Are you crossing the finish line in a race? Maybe you just had a baby. We might not always look our best after running a marathon or after hours of labor, but even if your hair or makeup isn't perfect, what you're seeing in these photos is that inner glow that radiates from your thoughts and lights up your face through your eyes.

This is the kind of beauty we want to have. It occurs when your brain is at its best and is focused on the joy and meaning of the moment. And it isn't always a spectacular event that creates this picture-perfect feeling. When you are engaged in anything that you are interested in or passionate about, your inner glow will shine from within.

Indulge in the New

It's never too late to become what you might have been.

—GEORGE ELIOT, NOVELIST

Every experience we have changes our brain. Even as you read this sentence, your brain is physically changing and making new connections. And what we now understand is that the richer and more stimulating your experiences are, the more profound these changes can be. Unfortunately many of us continue to just go through the paces of everyday life: work, kids, chores, bills, meals, rinse and repeat. Our brain slips into autopilot, and instead of forging new connections we use the same neural pathways again and again, like running in circles around a track. But our brain craves novelty, so when we are stuck in a rut we are boring our brains. And while you won't literally go brain-dead from boredom, you are depriving your brain of stimulating mental activity, which is essential for staying young and vibrant, in mind and in body.

The first step of your personal beauty/brain makeover is surprisingly simple and doesn't require medication, invasive surgery, or an enormous investment of time: I want you to open yourself up to five new experiences. Many studies suggest that the more we are engaged in stimulating activities, the less likely we are to develop dementia.

Indulging in new experiences is like sipping from the fountain of youth.

The stories below are based on women whom I have met in my personal life or in my practice. They have all fallen into a rut and need to Indulge in the New in order to experience more Beautiful Brain Days.

✦ As new parents, Ashley and her husband, both in their thirties, waited six months after their daughter was born before going out to a romantic restaurant. During dinner, however, the only thing Ashley talked about was "the baby." Her husband tried to change the subject several times, but somehow it always segued back to their daughter. Ashley used to have a wide range of interests, and her husband missed the engaging discussions they used to have, which made them feel more intimate. Ashley admitted that she has been so focused on motherhood that she felt she had nothing else to share, and that lately she hadn't read anything but parenting magazines.

✦ Pamela, a single workaholic in her forties, follows a daily routine that is as precise as a Swiss watch. She has lunch at her desk every day, and on weekends she orders takeout from the same restaurant, which she eats while she watches a rented movie. Although she earns a good salary working as an accountant, her job no longer offers the mental challenges that made it fun when she first started her job. She missed her college days, when she felt excited by her future and the endless possibilities that lay ahead. Pamela can't remember the last time she went out on a date.

✦ Marisol is an empty nester who has lived vicariously through her children for the past twenty-four years. Her friends tell her she's a great listener because she never talks about her personal life, mostly because she doesn't have one. She feels a void inside and has nothing to look forward to except the weekend phone calls from her kids. She and her husband rarely make love anymore, and she doesn't know what she can do to enjoy what should be a second honeymoon.

✦ After Katherine, a seventy-six-year-old widow, suffered from a stroke, she needed to walk with a cane. She used to be involved in many activities and organizations, but she is now embarrassed by her condition and rarely goes out with friends. They used to call to check in on her and ask her to join them for upcoming meetings and events, but she's made so many excuses about why she can't go that the phone has stopped ringing. Although her doctor reassured her that her memory was not affected by the stroke, she's been feeling mentally dull and forgetful lately.

Whatever your age or stage of life, your brain needs and pines for new experiences and stimulation to feel alive, active, and beautiful! Awakening your mind by indulging in the new will not only make you sharper, but it will also give you that boost of self-confidence you need to feel better about yourself and your life. You will experience an enhanced self-esteem that will extend to every facet of your life—including your sex life. It is a fact that boosting your self-esteem is a natural aphrodisiac! As you stimulate your mind, you'll stand a little taller, smile more often, and experience more joy in the world around you.

Transforming Bad Brain Days into beautiful ones begins by making simple changes in your routine, which can be anything from going to a museum during your lunch hour, to trying out a new recipe or listening to a new radio station. I know it sounds too simple, but even the smallest changes will begin to transform the way you think and the way you look and feel. Later I will help you to choose a Passionate Pursuit, a new endeavor that requires more effort, such as gardening, learning how to play an instrument, or mastering new computer skills. Keep in mind (pun intended) that the more you immerse yourself in a new activity and the more passionate you are about what you are doing, the greater the rewards.

CHANGE YOUR MIND

A wise man changes his mind, a fool never.
—Spanish proverb

Before we begin, I want you to understand what happens to your brain when it is exposed to new information. When we experience something new, the prefrontal cortex—the area of your brain that is constantly monitoring your environment—literally perks up. Think of this area of your brain as your personal CEO. It directs attention, makes decisions, reasons, and solves problems.

Working together with the hippocampus (your memory center; see sidebar on page 11), these areas fire up when the brain is presented with new stimuli and mental challenges. Because these parts of the brain age the fastest and are the most vulnerable to the ravages of Alzheimer's disease, we must keep them fit and strong throughout our lifetime. You can do this by challenging your mind with new activities and new opportunities to learn.

As with any new skill, the more you practice, the stronger your brain will become. For example, in a study conducted at the International University in Bremen, Germany, researchers taught healthy children and adults between ages six and eighty-nine how to juggle. The results showed that after just seven days of training, there was a measurable increase in gray matter in the area of the brain that processes visual tracking. Although the change was temporary, it clearly showed how our experiences can shape our brain.

In another German study, researchers did magnetic resonance imaging (MRI) scans on medical students before, during, and three months after their intensive studying for board exams. The MRIs showed a significant increase in the volume of the parietal lobes and the hippocampus. Even more remarkable is that three months after they stopped studying for exams, the med students' hippocampus continued to expand. Scientists now believe that this continued growth of the hippocampus is likely due to neurogenesis, the birth of new neurons that are stimulated by learning.

These studies show that we truly have the capacity to design and shape our brain. Our experiences, the choices we make daily, and the ways we use our brain ultimately determine its structure. Indulging in the new and challenging your mind optimize your brain's ability to reinvent itself.

I Remember It Well

When I was in high school my father gave me one of the most valuable books I ever read. It was called *The Memory Book* by Harry Lorayne and Jerry Lucas. It explains how to remember anything by tapping into the power of association and visualization. Throughout college, medical school, and even now, I use this memory system. To remember that the hippocampus is the memory center, for example, you need to form a mental picture that will stick. The word *hippocampus* makes me think of a "hippo" on a college "campus." Picture a huge hippo lying on its belly in the middle of the college quad. He is the center of attention, as the students must walk around him to get to class. Between his front feet he holds a list of facts that he is trying to commit to memory. He repeatedly taps the list against his forehead to force the information into his brain. If you visualize this scene, you too will never forget the hippocampus.

When I had to learn large volumes of information during medical school and residency, I would actually draw these scenes out in notebooks. I'll never forget the day I was reviewing my memory drawings as I often did while exercising on the StairMaster at the gym. A curious man on the machine next to me asked, "Do you write comic strips? I always see you studying cartoons."

REJUVENATE YOUR MIND

The adage "you can't teach an old dog new tricks" is patently false. A recent study by Dr. Karlene Ball revealed that subjects ranging in age from sixty-five to ninety-four performed better on cognitive tests when they were instructed on how to improve memory, reasoning, or speed. Even more impressive was the fact that two years afterward, the participants who had been trained still outperformed the control group, which did not receive instruction. The good news here is that even if you have neglected your brain for years it doesn't hold a grudge. It's never too late to learn something new, and there is no limit to what you can learn. Learning is like exercise—the more you do it, the stronger and smarter you get.

Thanks for the Memories—
the Hippocampus at Work

The brain's memory center, the hippocampus, is like a library. The hippocampus, like the librarian at the circulation desk, files and sorts information that comes in daily. If the librarian isn't at her desk, the new journals and newspapers don't get stored on the shelves or placed in the proper stacks. The library soon becomes outdated.

The files that were either shelved correctly or have been up in the stacks for years may still be available. However, the brain cannot stockpile new memories if the hippocampus is faulty.

When someone suffers from Alzheimer's disease, the hippocampus becomes riddled with amyloid plaques, and the brain cells in this vital structure die off. It's as if there is no librarian at the front desk, so memories are never stored, which is why people suffering from Alzheimer's disease have difficulty remembering new things or making new memories. Old memories, however, which were stored up years ago in the stacks located in other parts of the brain, are not affected until the disease spreads to other regions. This is why people with dementia might not be able to remember what they had for lunch but can recall the names of their elementary schoolteachers.

The hippocampus is special because it is one of the brain areas that can actually generate new cells. Many researchers believe that stimulating our memory circuits promotes neurogenesis, and that this new growth may protect us against memory loss. Once you understand that you have your hippocampus to thank for the formation of your memories, it's easier to appreciate the beauty of brain cell regeneration and the importance of keeping those circuits firing to maintain your mind's youthful vitality.

YOUR LIFE LEARNING CURVE

Our exposure to new experiences and new opportunities usually peaks when we are in school. After that, it's easy to get caught up in the routine of daily life, where we stop challenging our mind or giving it a workout. Take a moment now to consider your own life and what I call your Life Learning Curve. Draw a graph with your age on the horizontal axis, starting at birth, and extending to your current age. The vertical axis represents the amount of new information and mental challenges in your life.

Now, what does your graph look like? Depending on your learning trajectory, it should vary like the rise and fall of the stock market. Perhaps there are upticks in your graph when you moved to a new city or started a new job. But if you are like many of us, you are probably noticing some downward drifts. As we get older it's easy to get caught up in a routine way of living, which means a routine way of thinking. We tend to solve the same types of problems and are not challenged to use our brain in new ways. In addition, certain events deplete us of fresh ideas and experiences

Having children is one way we stay hooked into current trends and new technology. Children create a constant stream of novelty. So when the kids leave the house we lose a vital connection to this other world, causing our learning curve to plummet. For some mothers, their learning curves drop when they live vicariously through their kids and neglect their own needs and talents.

Other events, such as leaving or losing a job, divorce, or illness, can also make our learning curve dip. Whatever direction your Life Learning Curve is going in, it is within your power to reverse it or launch it even higher by tapping into the power of your mind. There is no need to surrender to life in a rut, because challenging your brain will revitalize you—whatever stage of life you are in at the moment!

Carol's Story

Carol, a fifty-six-year-old retired schoolteacher, told me that she thought she was "losing it." Over the previous six months she'd had trouble recalling words and, in particular, names. "It eventually comes to me," Carol explained, "but it is so embarrassing." The last straw was when she ran into a former student, a standout in her class, whose name she could not remember.

Although she had dreamed of retiring, she found herself not enjoying it as much as she thought she would. Carol lived alone in the home where she had raised her now grown children. She spent most of her time at home doing chores or small projects around the house. "I keep myself busy," she told me, with little enthusiasm.

After listening to Carol's story, I had a hunch that it was no coincidence that her symptoms began in the autumn, when she would normally be returning to the classroom. It was also not surprising that her symptoms progressed during the long New England winter, which isolated her even more by keeping her inside her home. After she performed perfectly on her neurologic exams, I told Carol that what she needed to do was to "indulge in the new."

Invigorated by a clean bill of health, she realized that she was not ready to retire, although the thought of returning to the classroom no longer inspired her. Instead, she indulged in her passions, which were gardening and flower arrangements. After taking a course in floral design, she began working at a local florist. She loved her work and excelled at making beautiful creations.

She went to flower shows and floral events and entered design competitions. She eventually teamed up with another designer, and together they opened a successful florist shop. Running her own business has filled Carol's life with a newfound passion and a wide circle of new friends. The next time I saw her, she had a sparkle in her eyes and an excitement in her voice that was once missing. It was clear that her prior concerns about memory loss had been long forgotten.

FIVE EASY INDULGENCES

The first step to achieving a Beautiful Brain Day is to open your mind to new ideas and experiences. It starts by being aware of the choices we make every day. If our life is filled with too many routines, we limit ourselves to narrow, sharply circumscribed mental pathways. I encourage you to venture out to create new brain pathways by making the choice to "indulge in the new." In our daily life we are surrounded by opportunities that can stimulate new ways of thinking. When you seek out new ways to change your brain, the process of transforming your entire being begins. You will notice a new gleam in your eyes that comes from being engaged in the world around you. Here are five easy changes to get you started.

1. Go for the "Aha!" Moment

Attempt to solve mysteries, riddles, and puzzles that present themselves in your daily life as well as those you find in books, magazines, and newspapers. Stay on top of the latest technological trends, from smart phones to new software programs so you and your brain can stay wired. Troubleshoot on your own the next time there's a glitch. Try performing mental calculations by being the one to divvy up a restaurant tab when you're dining out with friends. Estimate your grocery bill before you get to the cashier. Challenge yourself by getting "do-it-yourself" books or becoming a handywoman who can fix broken objects and make minor repairs around the house.

2. Read, Baby, Read

The fact that you bought this book means you already understand the value of reading, but you might not be aware of how it actually changes the brain on a physical level. As a uniquely human skill, reading not only expands your knowledge but also is a great workout for your mind.

When we read, precise eye movements smoothly course over the material. The visual system gears up as it is bombarded by multitudes of straight and curvy lines. Language areas switch into overdrive to identify and decipher symbols into meaning and context. The frontal lobes provide sustained attention and process the information, while the visual association cortex, otherwise known as the mind's eye, also gets a workout. The hippocampus and memory circuits are busy recording the new information flowing in. Through this incredibly complex mental activity we gain understanding and knowledge.

One of the best ways to open your mind to new ideas is to read every day. Keep up with current events by reading a daily newspaper or news blogs such as the Huffington Post, the Daily Beast, or Politico. The quality of the paper you read is important, so I recommend subscribing to the *New York Times* or the London *Times*. In fact, courses that prepare medical students for their rigorous board exams often recommend reading the *New York Times* because it is written in a more complex format than other newspapers. Clicking on a news story's hyperlinks is a great way to bring yourself up to speed on topics and issues that you don't understand and provides an endless source of information on topics that might spark your interest.

Browse a bookstore or newsstand and pick up a book or specialty magazine on something that interests you. If you feel there's not enough time in the day to read, do it in spurts while you are commuting, standing in line at the bank or supermarket, or right before you go to bed. Listening to audiobooks while you are commuting is another excellent way to keep your mind active.

3. Change It Up

Do you shop at the same venues, frequent the same nightspots, and travel to the same destinations? Are your weekends filled with a monotonous string of dinners and a movie? If so, now's the time to shake things up and explore some new activities. Check out local listings for some new things to do and different places to go. Going out to different types of restaurants, especially those where it's a challenge to pronounce the dishes, stimulates the brain by exposing you to new tastes and culinary experiences. Whether you live in a small town or a big city, there are auctions, fairs, museums, concerts, shows, and a variety of entertainments to choose from.

Whether you drive or walk, take a new route on your way home. It may take a little longer and you may even get lost, but you'll be doing your brain a favor by exposing it to different landmarks and landscapes along the way. In the process, you may discover a new art gallery or a funky boutique with great shoes.

And if you can't remember the last time you traveled outside your city limits, you must take a train, plane, or automobile to anywhere but where you are right now. It doesn't have to be far, as long as it's new. So if your vacations always involve a beach chair and a mai tai, spend your next holiday hiking, volunteering on a service trip, or going to museums instead.

4. Get Stylish

How long has it been since you've updated your look? Are you still wearing the same hair, makeup, and style of clothing that you wore five years ago? Search through magazines and online for fashions and styles that excite you. Check out new shops and salons in your area. Why not try that gorgeous haircut or color that you've admired on other women? Let your new look reflect your new outlook on life. Be adventuresome and creative as you discover your own chic style. Indulging in a new look is a fun way to break up your routine and give yourself a makeover from head to toe!

5. Be Pleased to Meet Someone

Striking up a conversation with someone you've just met can fire up your brain and open new avenues. Take advantage of the opportunities you have in your everyday life to start a conversation, such as while you are in the grocery store line or when you're clothes shopping. You never know what interesting people you might meet or how a total stranger can transform your personal or professional life. Maybe you will make a new friend, or that person might know someone who can help you find a job or, if you're single, a date. So take the initiative and make a habit of striking up a conversation whenever possible. If you are uncomfortable, as many are, with meeting new people, read Dale Carnegie's self-help classic *How to Win Friends & Influence People* or Diane Darling's *The Networking Survival Guide*. The more new people you meet, the more opportunities you'll find to learn new things.

Let Your Mind Blossom

Develop the art of contemplation and rediscover your brain's natural curiosity by asking questions. Whether you are watching a magnificent sunset or listening to politicians debate, ponder the information your brain is processing and pay attention to the questions that emerge. How are all those colors splashed across the sky? Is that senator really telling the truth? Take advantage of the many fabulous search engines and Web sites, including Google, Bing, AltaVista, Wikipedia, and Ask.com, to get the information you want. Never before has so much knowledge and expert advice literally been at our fingertips.

When you come across a word you don't recognize or something you don't know—find out. Go to www.dictionary.com to sign up for the Word of the Day, which will be e-mailed to you. This is a fun and effortless way to expand your vocabulary. You could also pay a visit to your local library or ask someone who is knowledgeable about a subject you are interested in to explain it to you.

Avoid the Brain Drain

Watching TV is a passive activity, so if you're spending more than two hours a day staring at the screen, your brain is essentially flatlining. Numerous studies have found that excessive TV watching is associated with sleep deprivation, depression, lower cognitive function, higher obesity rates, and a decline in overall physical health. If you want to make over your brain—that is, keep it sharp, efficient, and productive—then consider cutting back on the time you spend in front of the tube. How about reading instead?

YOUR INDULGE PRESCRIPTION

Now that you're expanding your brain's horizons through the Five Easy Indulgences, the new ideas and experiences you have will become a catalyst for even greater learning opportunities. But before you begin the next important step in your makeover, I want you to understand what is going on in your brain.

Mastering new skills and indulging in unique experiences are keys to a sharper memory and healthier brain. New information perks up the brain because it can't handle new ideas by using the old ways of doing mental business. It's like building a new bridge and reinforcing it with stronger cables.

This is how memories are made and knowledge is stored. New information uses brain circuits and neurons that are waiting to be developed. This happens every time you think and do things differently. New ideas and thoughts open new pathways, connecting the markedly different neighborhoods of the brain so that they all network in the labyrinth of complex information sharing. It's this process that leads to brain growth.

But to fully reap the benefits of neuroplasticity and achieve a complete beauty/brain makeover, a deeper commitment is required. You need to challenge your mind and make it even more robust by following my Indulge Prescription, which involves indulging in an activity outside your comfort zone—something you've always wanted to do but never pursued, such as learning Italian or knitting. Whatever the new activity, it should be something that you are passionate about.

Why Puzzles and Games Aren't the Best Brain Boosters

While puzzles that involve wordplay or numbers may provide some brain benefits, they can be socially isolating, and the skills you develop by doing them are relatively superficial and limited to that specific activity. Likewise, if you enjoy playing video games, your game scores might improve over time, but you're not learning a skill that can be put to practical use in your daily life. Moreover, your learning curve flattens with practice, as do the mental benefits.

A better way to challenge your mind is to pursue a new passion and life skill. For example, instead of spending countless hours doing Sudoku, try your hand at learning sign language or join a knitting group. Both the knowledge and skills you acquire can transfer to other facets of your life, such as volunteering to translate for the hearing impaired or being able to give homemade baby shower or holiday gifts. These kinds of passionate pursuits are "life skills" because they are practical as well as mind-enhancing talents. Learning new life skills will give you a sense of accomplishment and a feeling of satisfaction that you can't get from a video game. More important, developing life skills will expand your intellectual, social, and artistic horizons. Remember the Life Learning Curve you drew earlier? Unlike puzzles or mind-training games, the height of your learning curve for whatever endeavor you choose will be limitless.

PASSIONATE PURSUITS

Taking joy in life is a woman's best cosmetic.
—Rosalind Russell, actress

Now that you're inspired (and your brain is ready) to indulge in a new skill, you must pick your passion. It could be quilting, celestial navigation, or gourmet cooking. Whatever you choose, when you are passionate about something, your concentration is improved, time seems to fly, and you feel rejuvenated from head to toe. Your brain chemistry changes and your internal reward system kicks in. When we pursue activities that we enjoy, dopamine and other "feel good" neurotransmitters are released. High dopamine levels improve our concentration, make us feel good, and reinforce rewarding behavior, making it the perfect beautiful-brain learning elixir.

Artists, musicians, and writers often talk about the "high" they feel when they are creating a painting, composing a song, or writing a novel. Researchers become impassioned by the quest for information and the thrill of discovery. Athletes pushing themselves in their sport produce endorphins, which is another brain chemical that gives us a sense of well-being. It's a little like falling madly in love, only it's with a pursuit instead of a person.

But you don't have to be a lover, an artist, or an athlete to experience passion. You must simply discover what it is that excites you. Vincent van Gogh once said, "The best way to know life is to love many things." I believe this is also the best way to develop your mind. Ask yourself what makes you feel good and puts a smile on your face. Is there something that you've always wanted to do but never got around to? Chances are those dormant brain cells are still filled with desire and are poised to reconnect and grow.

And as you embark on your Passionate Pursuit, be sure to seek out the very best instructors and resources you can find. Think about the teachers from your past who inspired you. What was it about their teaching style or personality that clicked? What types of learning environments work best for you? The beauty of educating ourselves as adults is that not only do we become more interesting people, but we also get to call the shots. So pick the best mentors you can find who will inspire you to fulfill your dream. When we are infused with passion, our creative spirit and intelligence show in our face, our body image, and the way we present ourselves to the world. Passion is the radiant light that shines from within.

BE YOUR BRAIN'S PERSONAL TRAINER

Every brain is different, so before you start indulging in a new passion, it's important to consider what activities are best for your individual brain. What do I mean by this? The Passionate Pursuit you choose depends on which area of your brain you use most often and which area is weakest and in need of a workout. As you would with muscles that have atrophied from lack of use, it is better to exercise the area of your brain that is used *less* often.

Every part of the brain serves a different function, but the easiest way to think about how the brain works and how it is structured is to divide it into right and left sides or "hemispheres." In right-handed people, language lives in the left hemisphere, making this the dominant side. In left-handed people, language might reside in the right hemisphere, the left hemisphere, or both. Because more people are right-handed than left-handed, we generally refer to the "left brain" as the dominant hemisphere and, therefore, the home of language.

Our two hemispheres are tightly interconnected and work as a unit rather than as two independent systems, but there are some generalized differences. The left brain, in addition to having responsibility for language, serves as our analytical and logical side. When we're performing activities that require reasoning, mathematics, information sequencing, language, symbol recognition, reading, or writing, our left hemisphere is highly activated. It's working out.

Conversely, our right hemisphere is home to our visual and spatial talents. This hemisphere specializes in seeing the "big picture." Activities that push the right hemisphere into high gear include artistic and musical pursuits as well as those that require visual spatial skills, emotional perception, and facial recognition. Some researchers suggest that this is also where humor lives.

Though our two hemispheres work together seamlessly and every activity engages our brain as a whole, focusing on the areas of your brain that are the weakest can help you become your mind's personal trainer. If you are an accountant who spends your days crunching numbers, for example, your left brain is being challenged. Taking an art class would be an excellent way to stimulate your underused right hemisphere. Likewise, if you are an artist, actor, or dancer who regularly engages her right brain, you might want to learn a new language or become proficient with computers to strengthen your left hemisphere.

The following are some left brain and right brain makeover suggestions for Passionate Pursuits.

PASSIONATE PURSUITS
FOR THE RIGHT BRAIN

Tune In to Music

Studies done on professional musicians have found that the area of their cortex, the outer layer of the brain dedicated to finger movement and motor control, is highly developed. Learning to play a musical instrument is one of the best brain boosters out there because it stimulates a variety of brain areas. It challenges your auditory cortex to better discriminate sound. Reading music engages areas of the brain involved with visual processing and decoding. Even when we are just listening to music and not moving a muscle, the parts of the brain involved in movement coordination are firing away.

You can also enhance your musical makeover by taking courses in music theory or music appreciation, going to concerts, and performing in recitals for friends and family.

Marching to a Different Drummer

When Marina learned to play the drums at age fifty-nine, the decision to pick up this musical skill late in life was more than a fulfillment of a childhood dream. Marina, whose mother was a patient of mine, told me she wanted to take steps toward slowing down the aging process by keeping her brain healthy.

She had watched her mother suffer from Alzheimer's, and she wanted to do whatever she could to fight off the disease. When Marina told me later that she had taken up the drums, her face lit up with excitement. "I wanted to use a part of my brain I'd never used before, and drumming taught me how to do more than one thing at once," Marina said. "Plus, playing the drums is so much fun." Aside from expanding her brain, when she plays well, the reward center in her brain also lights up, giving her a sense of accomplishment.

Reap What You Sow

Gardening allows you to get in touch with your thoughts as well as with the earth. This relaxing activity "opens your eyes" by improving your visual perceptiveness. If you plant a hydrangea in your garden, for example, its unique leaf color and pattern will be encoded in your visual cortex. Once encoded, you will recognize it in a blink of a neuron the next time you see one, even when it's not in bloom, whether in a neighbor's front yard or in a public park. Memorizing the Latin and common names for plants is also a great memory workout. Your new appreciation for a plant's unique beauty will enhance memorization.

Gardening provides countless ways to cultivate your mind, from understanding plant biology to learning the art of landscape design. Join a gardening club, search the Web for information, take classes in horticulture, visit your local florist, and tour gardens and arboretums for ideas and inspiration. Watch your flowers and your mind blossom!

Become a Designing Woman

Learn how to knit, sew, or crochet. Challenge yourself with more complicated patterns or, better yet, create your own designs. These crafts enhance visual and spatial skills and provide a unique sense of accomplishment—not to mention the one-of-a-kind gifts you'll be able to create. So listen to this pearl (or purl) of wisdom and go make yourself a hat or sweater. Quilting is another time-honored art form that is not only challenging but also offers an excuse to meet regularly with your fellow quilters.

Act Out

Find a local theater group and perform in a local play or musical. Hone your skills by taking acting and voice lessons from a professional. You will gain a new awareness of body language and voice intonation as well as a new appreciation for the performing arts. Consider taking a literature course to study the classic playwrights or contemporary works that interest you. Watch plays and films to study our finest actors, including Meryl Streep, Halle Berry, Judi Dench, Penelope Cruz, Sean Penn, Denzel Washington, and Daniel Day Lewis, to name a few.

Become a Renaissance Woman

Indulge in the fine arts by learning how to draw, paint, or sculpt. You can also become an artisan by making pottery, prints, and jewelry. Whatever you choose, learn as much as you can about your chosen art form by taking classes and studying the masters. Expand your understanding of not only the history behind your artistic pursuit but also contemporary trends and techniques. Experiment with multimedia and new technology to make your art truly one of a kind. You never know where this could lead. I recently met a visual image artist, for example, who uses Fractiles (derived from mathematical equations) to create mesmerizing graphic forms. Attend shows, exhibits, and crafts fairs and subscribe to special-interest magazines to fully immerse yourself in your art.

Bask in the Laughter

Join an improv group or try your hand at stand-up comedy. Expose yourself to a variety of comedians by going to comedy clubs or watching Comedy Central. Read books by comedians who tickle your funny bone, such as Steve Martin, Stephen Colbert, Nora Ephron, and Chelsea Handler. Do some research on how they became successful and honed their craft. Practice giving humorous toasts at weddings and other special occasions.

PASSIONATE PURSUITS FOR THE LEFT BRAIN

Mind Your Money

Are you fascinated by stocks and bonds? Given the recent recession, who isn't nowadays? Joining an investment club is a surefire way to watch your knowledge of the market grow (and, who knows, maybe your portfolio will grow along with it). Watch *Mad Money* on CNBC, read books by Suze Orman, and subscribe to the *Wall Street Journal* to fill your mind with new information about the world of finance.

Did you know, for instance, that women are considered to be better overall investors than men? A study by the University of California at Davis found that women's portfolios gained 1.4 percent more than men's portfolios did. What's more, single women did even better than single men, with 2.3 percent greater gains.

Go to www.savvyladies.com to find a Savvy Ladies group in your area. Savvy Ladies is an organization that provides financial education to women. The founder, Stacy Francis, will assign an expert facilitator in your town to act as your investment sherpa and guide your group on its financial journey.

Parlez-Vous Français?

Numerous studies have shown that being bilingual is an excellent brain booster and protects against mental decline. While these studies looked at people who learned a second language in childhood, the latest research suggests that challenging your mind by learning another language will benefit your brain at any age.

To get an even bigger bang for your brain buck, find more than one way to increase your knowledge of a new language. If you are learning French, for example, in addition to taking a course at a local college or French institute, rent some French films, visit a country where they speak the language so you can practice and learn about the culture, take up French cooking, eat at French restaurants, listen to French singers, and read magazines and books written in French. The more ways you immerse yourself in your new skill, the better the brain benefits and the greater your joie de vivre!

Embrace New Technology

Steve Jobs, the founder of Apple, once described the personal computer as "a bicycle for the mind" that allows people to "explore as never before." Being computer savvy gives you access to a new world of information and knowledge, including what organizations you might like to join and events you might like to attend. Technology not only allows you to explore new worlds, but it also exercises your mind in the process as you learn new computer skills.

If you have not yet fully embraced high technology and all it has to offer, this should be at the top of your personal training program's to-do list. As we become more dependent on technology, it is crucial to stay on top of the latest gadgets, sites, blogs, software, and computer tools. Don't be discouraged if you haven't kept up with all the latest inventions and applications (called "apps").

Consider taking an adult education course on technology at your local college or library, or read up on how to get started. Your employer might even be willing to finance a course if you convince your boss that it will help improve your job performance. If you have children or teenagers who were weaned on technology and could program a computer by the age of three, ask them to teach you the basic skills.

For those who are already techno savvy, try learning HTML, Excel, Flash, Photoshop, Dreamweaver, InDesign, or another software program. You can practice your new skills by producing a book or designing a blog or Web site. The more you know about technology, the more plugged in you will be to the world, so get wired!

Become a Master Chef

Following a recipe requires logic and sequential processing. If you decide to specialize in a particular cuisine, try one that you are not familiar with. Start a gourmet club with a group of friends. Get a quality cookbook that explains the science behind food preparation—it is, after all, chemistry. Delve into nutrition, organic food, or the latest trends in slow food and buying local, and savor the new synapses that begin to simmer.

Bridge, Anyone?

Contract bridge requires a strong memory. It involves four players, paired off, with each player reading his or her partner's strategy by closely following what is played. Good players remember every card played and its significance for the team. Microsoft founder Bill Gates and investor Warren Buffett are both passionate bridge players; they recently started a fund to teach bridge in schools. Go to www .bridgeschool.com to learn more. If bridge sounds like something you might enjoy, I suggest joining a bridge club, reading up on strategies, and ramping up your game by challenging more advanced players.

Write Away

Have you dreamed about writing a book or magazine article? Hone your skills by journaling and reading quality literature. Consider getting a writing coach or forming a writing group with other aspiring authors. Book clubs are another great way to introduce yourself to genres and authors you might not have chosen on your own. Discussing literature with others will also expand your understanding and appreciation of the written word.

Optimize Your Practice Time

t's best to practice your newfound skill more frequently for short periods rather than less frequent longer periods. If you intend to practice one hour a week, for example, you will learn a new skill better by practicing three times a week for twenty minutes, instead of one hour-long chunk. This not only maximizes your brain's learning potential but also makes more productive use of your time.

HAVE MULTIFACETED PASSIONS

Whatever you choose to indulge in, consider a variety of ways to broaden your experience. Take classes, if possible, so you can improve your technique. Join organizations and blogs to stay connected with others who have similar interests. Sharing your passionate pursuits further boosts the brain benefits and your commitment level. Once you start sparking up your neurons and unleashing your mind's potential, you will likely find that one passion naturally leads to another. As you continue to indulge in your passions, you will find that, in the words of Mae West, "too much of a good thing is *wonderful!*"

Remember that the suggestions above are just that—suggestions— so feel free to come up with your own ideas. Maybe you've always dreamed about starting your own business or developing a fragrance. The possibilities for expanding your mind and your life are endless. As you open your mind to new ideas and engage in activities that are both challenging and fun, you will experience a new sense of self-confidence, fulfillment, and joy that will radiate from within. This is the transformative power of a beauty/brain makeover. Now get ready to "Rev Up Your Social Life"!

Rev Up
Your Social Life

*Life is partly what we make it, and partly
what it is made by the friends we choose.*

—TENNESSEE WILLIAMS

In this second step of your brain makeover I want you to introduce more friends, acquaintances, family, and fun into your life. An active social life is one of the keys to a beautiful brain and a beautiful you. Scientific studies consistently show that the more social we are throughout our lives, the less likely we are to suffer a decline in cognitive and motor skills as we age. Socializing is also associated with better health and fitness, which in turn gives us a more youthful appearance. This step will help you to understand how your brain is designed to communicate with others, and why indulging in new friendships will help keep your mind young and agile. And the more beautiful your mind, the better you will look! Revving up your social life involves:

+ Improving your social skills by being aware of
  the intricate link between your thoughts and facial
  expressions.

✦ Enlisting at least one friend as a Beautiful Brain Buddy
to join you in your journey to stimulate and rejuvenate
your mind.

✦ Enhancing your brain function by seeking out new
friendships and enriching old ones.

✦ Diversifying your social network so you can expose
yourself to new, mind-expanding ideas.

✦ Thinking about the relationships in your life that zap
you of your confidence and prevent you from reaching
your full potential.

✦ Ramping up your passion by meeting or reconnecting
with a romantic partner.

YOUR TALKATIVE MIND

Before you begin recruiting Beautiful Brain Buddies and making new
friends, I would like to explain how the mind helps us make social
connections in the first place. It might sound strange, but our brain
craves companionship. In fact, a significant portion of our brain is
dedicated to language—the primary way we communicate. Language
not only allows us to connect with others, but it also enriches our
personal experience by helping us to recall our past and to plan for
our future. It makes us uniquely human, because though other animals can certainly communicate and socialize (think about how your
dog lets you know it wants to be petted), they have yet to actually say
"Please rub behind my ears."

Remember the two brain hemispheres I described in the last step? Each plays an important role in communication. Our left hemisphere provides the words, while our right hemisphere imparts emotional meaning to what is being said. For example, if I said "It's snowing!" these words, which were produced in the left side of my brain, would be received and understood in *your* left hemisphere. But you wouldn't know whether I was excited or upset about the snow unless your right hemisphere also received the emotional cues in my facial expression and intonation from *my* right hemisphere. This nonverbal form of communication is called prosody. If I said "It's snowing!" with an upbeat tone of voice and with a delighted grin, you would not only be informed about the weather, but you might even guess that I love to ski!

Of course, most of us take our communication skills for granted, unless these neural pathways become compromised by a stroke, tumor, or other neurologic conditions. When this happens, neural pathways become blocked. In some cases, one can understand language but be unable to respond in turn. In other instances, someone will be able to speak fluently but won't be able to understand what is being said. Speech becomes what we call a "word salad"—a mixture of meaningless babble. Similarly, when prosody pathways are impaired, one might lose the ability to infuse emotion into words. Language becomes devoid of feeling and has a monotone pitch similar to that of the computerized voice on a GPS.

Other problems that might arise are an inability to interpret facial expressions or to decode emotional voice intonations. These kinds of impairments can also occur in what is called autism spectrum disorders such as Asperger's. This condition makes it difficult to bond with others because you might not be able to "get" a joke or to determine if someone is angry or ecstatic. Because autism spectrum disorders have become increasingly common, a tremendous amount of research has been done on social skills therapies. A variety of programs for both children and adults are available that are aimed at improving the ability to read emotions and enhance social interactions,

By understanding the role our brain plays in creating and interpreting language, we can fully appreciate the amazing feats that the mind performs every day.

FACE FACTS

Though expressing thoughts and emotions through language is a vital part of making social connections, numerous studies have found that nonverbal communication can be even more powerful than the spoken word. Arguably one of the most significant ways humans express their emotions is through facial expressions—especially with their eyes. And while we are able to control some of our facial and body language, our microfacial expressions (the subtle, fleeting muscle movements that reflect our thoughts) are involuntary.

Noted psychologist Paul Ekman, Ph.D., discovered that even when you try to hide your feelings and thoughts, they unconsciously flicker across your face. In his book *Emotions Revealed*, Dr. Ekman writes about how humans express seven universal emotions: anger, sadness, fear, surprise, disgust, contempt, and happiness. Experts are now using Ekman's Facial Action Coding System (FACS) to decipher which of the forty-three muscles of the face are working at any given moment, even when a person is unaware of it. All this can help us in our everyday lives because the better we are at understanding and interpreting these and other more subtle expressions, the better our social interactions will be.

Let's say you meet someone new and you're feeling nervous or unsure of yourself. You will probably plant a big wide grin on your face to show that you are open and accessible. Everyone fakes a smile now and then—maybe you even faked one today. But if we're not truly happy on the inside, our eyes won't come along for the ride. A genuine smile, in contrast, involves the tiny muscles around the eyes that reflect those happy thoughts in our brain that are involuntarily transmitted onto our face.

Fortunately, it is possible to smile authentically by changing our thoughts. Remember the song "Put on a Happy Face"? Dr. Ekman found that when we mimic a desired expression, we actually begin to feel the corresponding emotion. This is due to the intricate link between our facial expressions and the neural circuits that correspond to that emotion. In other words, by smiling (even if it's forced), we gently uplift our mood and actually feel happier.

Multiple studies confirm that happier people not only look more attractive, but they actually live longer. Positive people are less likely to suffer heart attacks, strokes, and pain from conditions like rheumatoid arthritis. Carnegie Mellon researchers found that people who express positive emotions are less likely to catch a cold or the flu than those who express negative emotions like anger, sadness, or stress. And we all know that the most attractive people are those who radiate good health and a sense of joie de vivre.

Facial Recognition

Our ability to recognize faces is an astonishing feat that we accomplish each day without giving it much thought. Consider for a moment all the faces that are stored in your visual memory: family, friends, colleagues, neighbors, acquaintances, historical figures, and celebrities. And what about the countless faces we have encountered over the years—from the cashier at your local supermarket to your kindergarten teacher? We recognize faces we know well, with glasses or without, with a new hairstyle or hair color, from multiple angles and perhaps, most remarkably, over time.

I experienced this firsthand when I ran into a friend whom I hadn't seen since the seventh grade. We had both changed dramatically over twenty-five years, and yet we recognized each other almost instantly. Even though neurologists do not fully understand how the brain creates this remarkable visual archive, we do know how essential this function is in our everyday social interactions. You can thank your brain for this ability to recognize faces, and celebrate it the next time you pass someone you know on the street.

The Truth about Botox

Botox, a neurotoxin that is literally toxic to nerves, is often used by dermatologists to erase facial lines and wrinkles. It works by blocking the release of neurotransmitters from the nerve endings connected to our facial muscles. Paralysis results when nerve transmission to the muscle is blocked. The problem with this cosmetic procedure is that it can also limit facial expressions, including the ability to display happiness or surprise. As a result, Dr. Ekman says the use of Botox can actually make someone look *less* appealing to others rather than more attractive. Consider this the next time you look in the mirror and notice some crow's-feet around your eyes. If you think of them as "laugh lines," these wrinkles will be reminders of all the good times you've had in your life!

THE EYES HAVE IT

You've heard the phrase "the eyes are the window to the soul"? To me, the eyes are the "window to the brain." In the introduction, I asked you to select some photos in which you look radiant. Take another look at those photos. Are you smiling broadly? Are your eyes lighting up your face? Now find another photograph where you were told to say "cheese" in order to force a smile. What do your eyes look like here? Does your face reveal that you were faking? As I mentioned earlier, your eyes reflect the true thoughts that were going on inside your head.

When I was taping the TV pilot for *Brain Talk with Dr. Marie,* a media coach asked me to picture various friends inside the camera lens. When I watched the tape later, it was fascinating to see how my eyes changed, depending on who was in my thoughts. For example, my eyes visibly softened when I envisioned my husband and became more animated when I pictured a friend who has a wonderful sense of humor.

Even the size of your pupils can reveal your innermost feelings. When we are attracted to someone, for instance, our pupils involuntarily dilate. It seems our brain wants to flood our visual circuitry with the image of our beloved by widening the portal of our eyes. Not surprisingly, because we are attracted to people who seem to like us, we subconsciously find people with large pupils more attractive. Studies have evaluated viewers' responses to the same photo of a person, one with artificially enhanced pupil size and one without. The photo with enhanced pupils is consistently rated as more attractive.

This is also why people find cartoon animals and babies so cute. In nineteenth-century Europe, women used a poisonous plant extract called belladonna (which is Italian for "beautiful lady") to dilate their pupils as a way to attract men. Unfortunately, belladonna also causes blurry vision, similar to when your ophthalmologist puts dilating drops in your eyes before an examination—not a particularly sexy side effect. Today photographers sometimes use the latest Photoshop technology to enlarge the pupils of magazine models to enhance their sexual attraction.

WHAT'S YOUR EYE-Q?

Psychologist Simon Baron-Cohen, Ph.D., author of *Zero Degrees of Empathy*, maintains that the female brain is predominantly hard-wired for empathy. Dr. Baron-Cohen developed a test that we have partially excerpted below to help determine how good we are at reading people's minds through the transom of their eyes. For each pair of eyes below, choose the word that best describes what the person in the picture is thinking or feeling. Even if you think you don't have a clue, just choose the one that "feels" right.

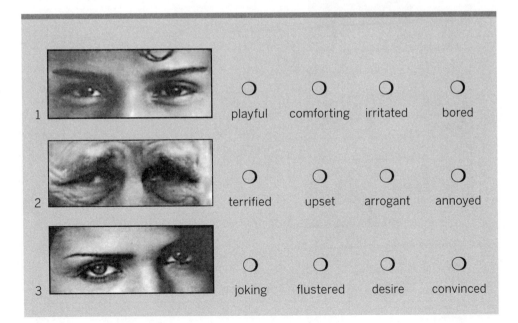

4
○ joking   ○ insisting   ○ amused   ○ relaxed

5
○ irritated   ○ sarcastic   ○ worried   ○ friendly

6
○ aghast   ○ fantasizing   ○ impatient   ○ alarmed

7
○ apologetic   ○ friendly   ○ uneasy   ○ dispirited

8
○ despondent   ○ relieved   ○ shy   ○ excited

9
○ annoyed   ○ hostile   ○ horrified   ○ preoccupied

10
○ cautious   ○ insisting   ○ bored   ○ aghast

THE CORRECT ANSWERS ARE: 1: playful   2: upset   3: desire   4: insisting   5: worried   6: fantasizing   7: uneasy   8: despondent   9: preoccupied   10: cautious

If you got many of these correct, you are good at decoding a person's facial expressions around their eyes. Most people surprise themselves by how well they do on this test. If you didn't do so well, you might want to practice "reading" people's emotions and tapping into your intuitive side. Women tend to find this easier to do than men. Honing your ability to intuit people's feelings through their eyes will increase your "emotional IQ." Of course, the better we know someone, the easier it is to read his or her nonverbal cues and expressions.

As an experiment, go back to the eye test and try mimicking the expression you see in the photos. You might find that you will begin to *feel* the emotion that is being expressed, which makes it easier to select the correct answers. As I mentioned earlier, in the same way that smiling can evoke feelings of happiness, this exercise further demonstrates the intricate neural link between our facial expression and our emotions.

Whenever we interact with others we involuntarily engage our emotional circuitry and mirror each other's feelings. I first discovered this phenomenon during my psychiatry rotation in medical school. We were told to "tune in to how patients made us feel" as they told their story. If we felt sad, chances are the patient was depressed; if we felt anxious, an anxiety disorder was likely.

The ability to read and copy other's emotions can be used to give your own face a "mind-lift." In recent years, neuroscientists have discovered what are called "mirror neurons," neurons that fire not only when we perform an activity but also when we observe others performing that activity. There is mounting evidence that mirror neuron systems play an important role in empathy and social interactions, allowing us literally to mirror the thoughts and feelings of others.

Picture yourself in the following two scenarios. In the first one, you are going out for breakfast and the server greets you with a genuine, friendly smile. Automatically you smile in return and your mood is uplifted. In the second scenario, the server is rude and surly, which triggers negative emotions within and a facial expression to match. If we're not careful, we could spread this negativity to the next person we encounter when we get to the office or return home. This is an example of mirror neurons at work.

By maintaining a pleasant and positive demeanor we can use these mirror neurons to make our facial expressions more appealing when we interact with others. Your inner contentment will give your face a mind-lift, and the people you encounter will "mirror" your mood without even realizing it!

Latisha's Story

Latisha, an attractive graduate student in her early thirties, had trouble meeting men and having long-term female friendships. She would go to parties with fellow students where she would connect briefly, but nothing ever seemed to click. Why would someone who had so much going for her have such trouble with her personal relationships? Without her realizing it, Latisha's expression was locked into a permanent frown. To make matters worse, she complained often about her troubles. It wasn't until a guy came up to her after class one day to ask "What's the matter—did your best friend die?" that she realized that her unhappiness was being broadcast on her face, which acted as a caution sign to anyone who dared approach.

After that, she made a concerted effort to think more positively and to smile, even if she wasn't feeling so cheerful on the inside. Eventually Latisha got the kind of attention she desired, her social life improved, and the happiness that she now expressed on her face was generated from a real feeling of contentment.

Mind-Reading Exercises

The following exercises will help you strengthen your observational skills.

✦ Ask a Beautiful Brain Buddy to sit directly across from you without uttering a word for three minutes. You can use a cooking timer for this exercise. During this exercise ask your friend to relive an emotionally laden event in his or her mind's eye. This can be anything—a wedding, birth, graduation, getting a flat tire on the highway. No gestures are allowed. See how well you can read your friend's expressions. Now switch roles. Afterward, compare your impressions and reveal what you were thinking about.

✦ As you become more confident of your skills, try extending your powers of observation to those you encounter throughout the day. For fun, subtly study the facial expressions of your fellow commuters on the bus or train, or the people you see standing in line at the bank. By simply focusing more attention on others, you will experience a deeper sense of connection with those around you, and most likely, with the help of mirror neurons, they will feel the same in return.

◆ Ask someone to videotape you while you are engaged in a five-minute interview with your Beautiful Brain Buddy. You can also use a tripod; make sure that the camera is taking a close-up of your face. Have your friend bring up hot-button topics, such as politics, family, or religion, that will evoke an emotional response. Next, play back the tape with the sound off and observe your expressions. Can you tell when you were speaking about something that made you upset? What does your face look like when you are pleased? What kinds of expressions do you use?

If you find that you are frowning or are blinking nervously, you can give yourself a natural face-lift and change the image that you present to the world by changing your thoughts. We'll talk more about this in Step 5, Make Over Your Mind.

SMART DRESSING

Victoria Billings clearly understood the neural link between how we feel and how we look when she remarked, "Any garment that makes you feel bad will make you look bad." Even if we wear a Versace creation with a knockout pair of Manolos, if our dress needs constant readjusting or our feet are pinched in agony, we will never look our best. Our eyes and our gait will reveal the truth of the discomfort in our feet and the annoyance of ill-fitting clothing. And although others may not know why we appear uncomfortable and distracted, they will nonetheless pick up on these negative vibes. Wearing clothes and shoes that both *look* good and *feel* good is the key to looking your best.

CONTAGIOUS EMOTIONS

Our moods and our happiness are strongly influenced by those around us. Nicholas Christakis, a professor of medical sociology at Harvard Medical School, and James Fowler, a political scientist at University of California, San Diego, have done fascinating studies on social networks showing that emotions are contagious. After tracking the relationships of more than five thousand people for decades, they concluded that both happiness and unhappiness are infectious. Fortunately, happiness spreads more readily than unhappiness. Knowing someone who is happy makes you 15.3 percent more likely to be happy yourself. And what's really fascinating is if your friend has a friend who is happy, even if you don't know them, your odds of happiness are increased by 9.8 percent! In other words, happiness ripples through social networks. The happiest people were those at the center of large social networks.

Similarly, negative emotions can also become viral. Any parent who has ever worried that their child is hanging out with the "wrong" crowd understands the problem of negative influences. The same holds true for adults. Is there someone in your life who drags you down? Are there people who you would like to spend less time with or stop seeing entirely? Chances are they fall into the "toxic" relationship category, which is someone who leaves you feeling drained, exhausted, and gasping for air. When a person is negative, you process those comments in your brain, which changes your brain chemistry for the worse. This doesn't mean you must give up on someone every time he or she says something negative, but be aware of the dynamics that are going on in your relationships.

I realize that cutting people out of our lives is not an easy thing to do, especially when a family member is the source of the problem. If this is the case, you might want to try changing the relationship through therapy or by gently letting that person know that their pessimism is upsetting to you. If you can't change the dynamics of your relationships for the better, then you can gradually cut back on the time you spend with them. Knowing when to end a friendship isn't easy and can be a heartbreaking experience, especially if you remember the good qualities that initially attracted you to that person. But as difficult as this might be, a toxic relationship creates stress in your life and in your brain.

Ultimately when we are with people we like, people who are happy, supportive, and make us feel good about ourselves, the positive emotions they produce are reflected on our face. Truly enriching relationships are mutually beneficial. Our friends will internalize and project these positive emotions back to us, multiplying the rejuvenating benefits. It's a win-win situation all around. Spending time with people who boost our spirits is like a trip to the spa. At the end of the day we feel physically, emotionally, and mentally uplifted.

Toxic Relationship Quiz

Answer the questions below to see if you have a "frenemy" in your life. And while other people's behavior can negatively impact our brain chemistry, you can also use this test to examine your own role as a friend. If any of the following sound more like you than like someone you know, it's time to change the messages that you are sending to yourself and to others.

Does your friend pretend to be supportive and concerned with your well-being while shooting down every new idea that excites you?

INSIGHT: This is the classic Two-faced friend who will come up with a hundred reasons why registering for that continuing education course you always wanted to take wouldn't work. She is the type who believes misery loves company, so your happiness will only remind her of how unhappy she really is.

Is there someone in your life who always sees the proverbial glass half-empty?

INSIGHT: The Pessimist is someone who will claim that she was passed over for a promotion because the boss is sleeping with a co-worker, or that it's no use dating because all the men out there are either married or gay. People who blame outside forces for personal failures are bound to live out their self-fulfilling prophecy of doom and gloom.

When you are with your friend, are you more apt to eat, drink, or spend too much?

INSIGHT: While the Addictive friend might be fun to be with, engaging in anything to excess will leave you feeling empty (or broke) when you crash out or cash out at the end of the day or night. Addictive person-alities often mean well, but it's best not to see them that often.

Does your friend talk incessantly about herself and rarely ask about what's new in your life?

INSIGHT: The Narcissist is the person who is always asking for favors but never seems to reciprocate. She lives in a bubble of her own private universe in which she is front and center. Narcissists are not likely to change into loving, caring persons, because the person they love and care about most is themselves.

When you go to a restaurant, is your friend always unhappy with the food and service and feeling that she is constantly being ripped off?

INSIGHT: Complainers are some of the most annoying people to have around, because they tend to snap at waitstaff and send back food as a way to exert their power over others. Complainers feel justified when things go awry, because it only proves their belief that everyone else is incompetent.

SOCIALIZE YOUR MIND

One of the most effective things we can do to maintain a beautiful mind is to stay connected with others. It's a surprisingly simple prescription, and study after study has shown that socializing, be it with friends, family, neighbors, colleagues, or caregivers, can help stave off dementia and the loss of motor skills as we age. Here are just a few of the most recent findings:

✦ The nearly decade-long 2009 Rush Memory and Aging Project found that elderly participants who had the least amount of social contact had a 40 percent increased risk of death and a whopping 65 percent increased risk of developing disabilities.

✦ A three-year study of more than two thousand women ages seventy-eight and older, which appeared in the 2005 issue of the *American Journal of Public Health*, concluded that larger social networks have a protective influence on cognitive function among elderly women.

✦ According to a study published in the 2009 issue of *Neurology*, middle-aged people who lived isolated lifestyles were more prone to cognitive decline as they age.

There is no question that surrounding ourselves with people who nurture and encourage us, support our dreams, and open our minds to new ideas is crucial to maintaining a vibrant brain. The healthier your relationships are, the more you infuse your mind with a bounty of positive energy. This positive energy will attract others to you like a magnet, further enhancing your beautiful brain benefits.

Here are a few suggestions for enhancing your social life and your social brain:

✦ **Be genuinely interested in others.** Take your conversations to a higher level by being curious about what makes others tick. What are people passionate about? What gives them that inner glow that lights up their eyes when they talk? This kind of enthusiasm and joie de vivre is the difference between a dull and a memorable interaction. If the person you are talking to is reticent about revealing her personal passions, make it a challenge to see if you can light up that sparkle in her eyes.

✦ **Talk about your new indulgences.** If you followed my advice in the previous step, you are now indulging in new activities and Passionate Pursuits. Look at these activities as a way not just to enhance your knowledge and learning but also to expand your circle of friends. These experiences should supply myriad topics for discussion. The more activities you are engaged in, the more exciting and interesting you will become and the easier it will be to attract friends.

✦ **Be aware of what's going on in the world.** If all you talk about is your work, your kids, or the hassles of the day, your brain (and companion) will get bored. You should read a news-paper every day, or at the very least watch the news, so you are informed about what is happening in the world. Discuss an article you read that sparked your interest or some new technology you've recently discovered. Memorizing information or stories to share with others is a meaningful way to challenge your memory. You may even want to keep a list of interesting ideas, stories, and experiences to help prod your memory.

✦ **Challenge your old ideas.** Challenge some of the views and assumptions that you've held on to for years. If we spend our time exclusively with those who agree with us, we are not challenged to think outside our personal box—and boxes are confining. Don't be afraid to share your views on politics, art, education, the environment, and parenting styles. Listen to as many viewpoints as possible and engage in healthy, mind-expanding debates. Exposing your brain to fresh ways of thinking will fire up new neural pathways as you analyze what the other person is saying. A brain that isn't stimulated by new thoughts is limited to thinking along routine pathways. In contrast, a brain that is open remains far more young and flexible with each influx of new ideas.

✦ **Learn from those around you.** Knowledge doesn't come only from books or schools (although I heartily encourage both!). Talking to others and exchanging information is another fun way to learn and to enrich your brain. Your neighbor might be able to teach you how to tune up your car, for example, or a culinary friend can show you how to make homemade pasta. There is a treasure trove of fascinating people out there who can elevate and expand your mind by simply sharing their expertise.

✦ **Become multicultural.** The more diverse your social network, the more benefits you will reap. Making friends with people who have different ethnic backgrounds and religions will open up your mind to new perspectives and expose you to other traditions and cultures. Forging friendships with someone for whom English is a second language is a good exercise for the brain. It might be difficult to understand them at first, but over time it will become easier to communicate as you learn about their culture and adapt to their accent, facial expressions, and body language.

✦ **Become multigenerational.** Although most of us tend to stick with people who are around our same age, I highly recommend that you reach out to people who are both younger and older than you are. In the same way that a multigenerational workforce benefits companies, having friends that span different generations will empower your mind. Consider how much we can learn from young people—they provide a unique window on the world, from pop culture to the latest technology. Similarly, the experience and wisdom of older individuals enrich our understanding of ourselves and the world around us.

✦ **Network.** Networking is another great way to increase your social circle. If you are a mom, you are likely to ask another mother if she knows of a good pediatrician in town. Similarly, whether you're looking for a hairstylist or a new computer, to get the best recommendation, it helps to know someone with expertise in that area. It's all about networking, and it's not just for gathering reliable information and making business connections; it's also an excellent way to make new friends.

✦ **Join support groups.** Studies show that group support is one of the most effective ways to successfully change behavior. This is why I asked you to select a Beautiful Brain Buddy to ensure that your social network is strong and supportive as you continue your quest for a better brain. You might also want to take advantage of support groups for other areas of your life that you wish to improve. Whether it's in AA, or in a cancer survivors or eating disorders group, finding people who are struggling with similar issues is an excellent way to find new friends who will be helpful, caring, and sympathetic. Ask your doctor or clergyperson, or search the Internet for a support or therapy group in your area that deals with your particular issue.

✦ **Try public speaking.** If you feel intimidated when meeting new people or you are afraid of speaking in front of large groups (and who isn't?), consider joining Toastmasters International, a nonprofit organization with clubs around the world that helps members practice and hone their communication skills in a nonjudgmental, positive setting. Go to www.toastmasters.org to find out more.

✦ **Join a book group.** Book groups are wonderful social events, and you might end up reading something you wouldn't have chosen on your own. Discussing books with others adds another dimension to the reading experience through the exchange of different ideas and interpretations. Start your own book group by gathering friends together, or go to your local bookstore or library to see if you can join one that is accepting new members. Challenge yourself by selecting books that you wouldn't ordinarily read for an extra brain boost.

✦ **Host monthly "salons."** Salons (not the hair kind) were big in seventeenth- and eighteenth-century France as a form of entertainment and as a way to increase one's knowledge through high-minded conversation. Invite your guests to bring an interesting article to discuss, something they've written themselves, or an instrument they can play. If you don't have anything to contribute that night, just sit back and soak in the creativity of those around you.

✦ **Have a regular girls' night out.** Get-togethers with friends don't have to be brainy in order to stimulate the mind. My girlfriends and I throw monthly facial nights where we sit around with our mud masks while talking about our careers and personal lives. One of my friends is an entrepreneur who is launching a new hair products line (thus, the facials). Another woman is an Austrian opera singer, and another started an art program for inner-city teens. They are amazing, fascinating women who range broadly in age, and our conversations are lively and fun. As my friend Linda, a teacher, remarked, "Something tribal and uninhibited happens when women gather together wearing mud masks." If facials aren't your thing, find another activity such as poker, bridge, quilting, or whatever it is you enjoy where you and your most interesting friends can have a girl fest.

✦ **Become a mentor.** Offer to mentor the younger employees at your job or others with whom you share a common career interest or hobby. I love working with the young residents at the hospital where I work. They keep me on my toes in terms of the latest medical information and technology because they are so bright and cutting edge. Mentoring relationships are often mutually beneficial and enjoyable because they are both emotionally and intellectually rewarding. They are also less complicated than our usual family and work relationships.

✦ **Volunteer.** This is a great way to meet others while dedicating your time to a cause that you believe in. Volunteer work can also serve as a springboard to discovering a new career. Not to mention, the people you meet are bound to have a big heart!

LOVE—THE BRAIN'S FAVORITE ELIXIR

Why do we say "I love you with all my heart," when the heart has nothing to do with it? Instead, we should be saying, "I love you with all my brain." And while poets, musicians, and artists have been celebrating love for centuries, neuroscientists are singing its praises because we know what a powerful elixir love is for the brain. When we fall in love, for example, dopamine, a "feel good," energizing neurotransmitter, appears to play an important role. Arthur Aron, a researcher at SUNY Stony Brook, performed brain MRI scans on people who had recently fallen in love as they gazed at photos of their beloved and of someone for whom they had neutral feelings. He found that areas of the brain rich in dopamine-releasing neurons lit up with activity only when the picture of each person's loved one was being viewed.

Dopamine is a multifaceted neurotransmitter that has many functions in the brain affecting behavior and cognition. It is believed to be a key player in our inner reward system, providing a natural high that improves concentration and drive. Helen Fisher, Ph.D., an anthropologist who has done extensive research on what happens to the brain when we are in love, concludes that romantic love is not an emotion but a "motivation" or drive that is fueled by our brain's reward system. In other words, our quest for romantic love is similar to the brain's natural drive for food, water, and sex. Love can be so addictive (thanks to the dopamine buzz) that the loss of it, Fisher says, can trigger the same kind of craving as a withdrawal from cocaine or cigarettes.

Fortunately for those who have been in long-term relationships, a natural dopamine high can be long lasting. Recent data presented by Drs. Arthur Aron and Bianca P. Acevedo revealed that romantic love in the later stages of a relationship shares many of the same intense qualities of newfound love. They studied ten women and seven men who claimed to still be in love after twenty-one years of marriage. When these volunteers were shown pictures of their partners, their fMRI (Functional MRI) scans lit up in the dopamine-rich areas of their brains. Even more encouraging was the fact that other areas of the longtime married brains ignited too, such as those associated with oxytocin, a hormone and neurotransmitter that evokes feelings of contentment and is believed to be important in attachment and bonding.

Although we're a long way from understanding the neurochemistry of love and romance, love appears to keep our brains and bodies healthy. A Finnish study of 1,449 midlife subjects found that those participants who did not have partners were three times as likely to develop cognitive impairment as those who had a loved one. There is also evidence that people in loving relationships are healthier than those who are not. That's the conclusion of a study that appeared in the *Annals of Behavioral Medicine*, where researchers found happily married people had lower blood pressure than singles. Of course, this doesn't mean that marriage alone is the ticket to better health. According to that same study, unhappily married participants fared the worst.

Another theory for these findings is that people who are in love tend to take better care of themselves and their bodies because they want to look good for their companions. Whatever the reason, the bottom line is that the more love and passion you have in your life, the better it is for your health. To that end, see the suggestions for igniting and reigniting your passionate self that begin on page 59.

Social Preening

Have you ever noticed that when we're having a bad hair day, we tend to avoid social interaction and duck into a crowd, hoping to go unnoticed rather than interact with others? Conversely on days when we've taken the time to look our best, we have that extra spring in our step and we're more likely to go out of our way to say hello and engage in conversation. And on these days, we not only look good because we're well groomed; more important, we *feel* good about the way we look, which gives us that "extra" glow from within. Taking the time to look our best is time well spent.

The Sensual Mind

Research in a new field of study called "embodied cognition" reveals that the brain can be extremely sensual. In a recent Yale University study, forty-one college students were divided into two groups. Group A was asked to hold a cup of hot coffee, and Group B was told to hold iced tea. The students were then asked to evaluate the personality of an imaginary individual based on a packet of information. The study found that the students who held the warm beverage were far more likely to judge the fictitious person as warm and friendly than those who held the iced tea.

Does this mean singles would have a better chance of making a love match over a steaming cup of hot chocolate than over a cold beer? In any case, studies like these show that incoming sensory information and environmental stimuli can influence our perspectives. So if you want to make a good first impression, try making your surroundings warm and fuzzy the next time you go out on a date.

PURSUING PASSION

✦ **MySpace or yours.** Blogs, Facebook, and MySpace have transformed the way we socialize, and online dating services like eHarmony and Match.com are now the easiest way to fill up your social calendar. If one of your new indulgences is volunteering for a political campaign, for example, check out political blogs and message boards to connect with others through a lively exchange of ideas. Treat online forums as you would a real-life gathering by never posting anything you wouldn't say at a party. Not only does what you write online reach a wider audience, but it also can go embarrassingly and permanently viral. Make sure to use a picture or avatar that expresses your personality and that you make thoughtful and frequent posts so you become a regular where everybody knows your screen name.

✦ **Your brain matters.** Keep a log of interesting stories you've heard, articles you've read, and movies, books, or events that you've enjoyed so you can flaunt your brain matter by having interesting topics to talk about when you are out on a date or at a social event. Review your journal before you go on a date to remind yourself of the talking points.

✦ **Use your new indulgences as a way to find potential love interests.** Take advantage of the fact that your Passionate Pursuits will boost your self-confidence and joie de vivre, which in turn will naturally boost your libido. Sharing an interest that you are passionate about with someone else can be a powerful aphrodisiac!

✦ **Practice the art of mingling.** The next time you're at a party or social event, take advantage of all the potential love interests who have gathered in one place just for you to meet! Don't spend the evening talking with the friend you came with—make it a point to meet at least two new people before you leave. The best way to enter a conversation in progress is to ask the host to introduce you to someone you want to meet, or gracefully break into a group of more than two people talking and wait for an opportunity to introduce yourself or make a comment about what's being said. Larger groups are easier to enter than deuces because two people are more likely to be engaged in an intimate conversation.

✦ **Don't be afraid to get set up.** Your friends and family know you best and want the best for you, so trust them to at least try to play matchmaker for you.

✦ **Throw a passion party.** The best way to guarantee that you will feel comfortable at a party is to throw your own. Have a dinner or cocktail party and ask each guest to bring someone else you don't know to help widen your circle of eligible partners.

Sex on the Brain

Has your sex life lost its luster? Or maybe you've yet to experience the much-touted joys of sex that we see in the movies, on TV, or online. If so, you are not alone. As many as 50 percent of women report having some kind of sexual problem, and if you factor in dissatisfaction the number is even higher. Yet few women ever seek help due to modesty, embarrassment, or simply resignation. The good news is that your brain can help you enjoy healthy and satisfying sex that will rejuvenate your body as well as your marriage or relationship!

How? As a neurologist, I can tell you that your primary sexual organ is between your ears. Your brain plays an integral role in desire and arousal. Try *thinking* about something or someone who turns you on and chances are you will start to feel something physically. Via neurotransmitters and hormones, these thoughts are sending messages from the brain throughout your nervous system that get you sexually aroused.

Once again, it is that feel-good chemical dopamine and other arousing neurotransmitters that are surging through your brain. Whatever the object of your desire, these rejuvenating neurotransmitters light up areas deep within the brain, triggering feelings of pleasure and reward. You feel a rush, and your heartbeat quickens. Attraction is also a powerful drug. When you see someone you think is sexy, the brain stem also gets into the act, releasing phenylethylamine (PEA), which speeds up the flow of information among nerve cells.

Unfortunately, there are many factors that can be a sexual buzz kill. Depression, child care, stress, and anger with a partner can put a damper on your sex life. Medications such as antidepressants, antihistamines, hormonal preparations, and the birth control pill, which alter brain and nerve activity, can also snuff out our desire. Other conditions, including diabetes, excessive drinking, and vaginal dryness, which occurs after menopause and makes intercourse painful, can also have a negative impact.

Whatever the cause for your flagging desire, the first step toward enjoying a healthy sex life is to speak with your doctor. Once you identify the underlying cause, you can start working on improving your love life. There are lubricants on the market that will help with vaginal dryness. Exercise, the Relaxation Response (see Step five), massages, and hiring babysitters can all help alleviate stress. And speaking of sex on the brain, try sharing your erotic thoughts with your partner so you can fire up your neurons and get neurochemicals and other things flowing.

Sexual activity not only revs up your heart rate, but also gives your body and your brain a rejuvenating workout. In the process, the increased blood flow beautifies your skin (aka "afterglow") and gives you that extraspecial, alluring sparkle in your eye!

RENEWING PASSION

✦ **Surprise your brain.** In the same way the brain is programmed to pay attention to new things, it also loves surprises. The unexpected can be a turn-on, especially when couples have been together so long that they can finish each other's sentences. Consider both of you packing your bags and buying tickets to a romantic destination for a weekend getaway. If you can't afford a minivacation, surprise him with tickets to a concert or reservations at a restaurant you've never been to before. Surprises like these will delight and light up your partner's romance circuits.

✦ **Make a pact to reconnect.** It's easy for couples to become world-weary, due to work, children, financial worries, and other stressors, so sometimes you have to schedule spontaneity. Try making every Friday night your turn to do whatever you want, and every Saturday will be your partner's turn. Be sure to shake it up by being adventurous and creative with your plans.

✦ **Shut off the electronic devices.** Late-night TV, cell phones, iPods, and other devices that keep us wired also make us tired, so shut down all your electronics, temporarily, so you can re-boot your love life and enjoy a real laptop for a change!

✦ **Go to a hotel or motel, even if it's somewhere in your hometown.** There's nothing more exciting than the idea of "il-licit romance" with your partner and a change of venue. It's good for your brain as well as for your love life.

✦ **Indulge your partner.** Share your brain makeover with your partner. Invite him to try new activities and pursuits with you. Encourage him to explore new interests on his own. At the end of the day, you both will have more to share with each other.

✦ **Indulge each other's desires.** Have you always wanted to take tango lessons? Maybe your partner has dreamed of white-water rafting. Whatever is on your bucket list, now is the time to indulge! The same goes for your bedroom routine. Like tak-ing a different route home, try going down a different path sex-ually and see where that leads. Ask your spouse to indulge you in your secret desires and do the same for him. As you know, novel activities stimulate dopamine release, the same neu-rotransmitter that gets activated when couples first fall in love. Indulging in new things and unusual sensual delights will essentially stimulate your brain chemistry, making sparks fly anew. And in doing so, you will share a new level of intimacy.

GET READY TO PAY YOUR BODY SOME MIND

As important as new indulgences and cerebral celebrations are, to fully enjoy your newfound friends and passions, you need a healthy brain and body. Most of us are aware of the mind-body connection, and I've explained a bit about how our thoughts can positively change the way we look and feel. But not as many people are aware of the "body-mind" connection, which is how our body impacts our mind. This is why the next step in your brain makeover will tell you what you need to know about staying in good physical condition, and what you need to ask yourself and your doctor so you can be in the best possible shape from head to toe.

Mind Your Body

*The body is your temple. Keep it pure
and clean for the soul to reside in.*

—B. K. S. IYENGAR, GURU

NATALIE'S CAUTIONARY TALE

By the time Natalie was in her forties she was no longer the 130-pound head-turner she once was in her twenties. In fact the last time she dared step onto a scale it topped 175 pounds, which she knew was not only unattractive but also unhealthy. But with the kids off to college, she found herself watching more television to help fill the time in her now empty nest. As she grew larger, she began caring less about the way she looked and gave in to her cravings, especially for salty chips, soda, and sweets.

She couldn't remember the last time she went for a checkup, telling herself that, except for being fat, there was nothing seriously wrong with her. Or was there? She often felt light-headed and was unusually tired by the end of the day. She couldn't put her finger on it, but she knew something was wrong. Was she depressed? After all, her mood was low and she had no desire for sexual intimacy. She also had an unquenchable thirst, which was why, she thought, she made so many trips to the bathroom. When she mentioned these symptoms to her husband, he convinced her to see a doctor, if only to alleviate her concern.

After performing a physical exam, Natalie's doctor thought she might be suffering from "metabolic syndrome." Her large waist circumference and her high blood pressure were the first clues. Subsequent blood tests revealed that her blood sugar was high and that her cholesterol and triglyceride levels were in an unhealthy range, confirming the diagnosis. If left untreated this combination of ailments wreaks havoc throughout the body, causing every organ system, including the brain and even our skin, to age faster. Metabolic syndrome, which is common in middle-aged women, can make us look and feel older than our years both inside and out.

Fortunately, through a combination of medication, a healthier diet, and regular exercise, Natalie was able to normalize her blood sugar, cholesterol, and triglyceride levels. She lost most of the weight she had put on over the years, and her blood pressure returned to normal. Eventually she no longer needed medication. And the best part was she felt a renewed sense of well-being. She had more energy than ever, her libido returned, and her husband said she looked like that sexy woman he fell in love with in college.

What Natalie discovered, and what I want everyone to understand, is that you need to listen to your body, which speaks to you through your brain. Your brain orchestrates every organ throughout your body via chemical messengers in the blood called hormones and through the nerves that extend from the brain and spinal cord. In turn, your body ensures that the brain has the proper supply of oxygen and nutrients to keep it running smoothly. When your body is out of tune, so is your brain, which then directly influences your moods, motivation, desires, energy level, and how you look. So in order to think, feel, and look your best, your internal organs must work together with your brain as one remarkable, high-functioning system.

The other advice that I hope you take away from this step is that a visit to your doctor can not only improve your life, but it can also *save* your life. In Natalie's case it was metabolic syndrome, but many women are at risk for heart disease, cancer, and a host of other illnesses that can be prevented or at least treated. This section is about how to "mind your body," which you should do with the same attention and loving care that you give to your family and loved ones.

TAKING CHARGE OF YOUR BRAIN

You can take charge of your brain and your body by taking care of your health. I've always thought that the Syms clothing store slogan, "An educated consumer is our best customer," should be applied to health care. Like Natalie, knowing as much as you can about any medical conditions that you might have, and learning what you need to do to keep yourself in the best shape possible, will ultimately empower you. So give yourself a pat on the back for reading this book, because you are obviously someone who cares enough to learn about what you can do to keep your brain and body in peak condition!

It all starts with a visit to your doctor. Your advocate and guide through this process should always be your personal physician, so it is vital that you find one whom you trust and with whom you feel comfortable. Don't feel as though you must stay with a doctor if it isn't a good fit. Over the years, many patients have told me that they find it difficult to talk with their primary care doctor or they believe their concerns are not being properly addressed. If you feel this way, it's time to make a change. Keep in mind that you have a choice about whom you see. Use your social network to find a doctor with whom you can comfortably talk and ask questions. Finding a doctor who will be supportive and actively involved in your health care is one of the best time investments you can make.

TALKING TO YOUR DOCTOR

Remember that your doctor is there to help you, not to judge you, so be open and honest when talking about your health and lifestyle. Here is a checklist that will allow you to get the most out of your visits:

✦ Make a list of questions, symptoms, and concerns before you go and take notes during your consultation so you can go over what was said.

✦ Consider taking a friend or family member with you—he or she can bring up questions you may have forgotten to ask, write down the answers to your questions, or assist you in remembering what was important.

✦ Tell your doctor how you are feeling and about any medical concerns. Don't be embarrassed to mention problems with libido, sexual dysfunction, anxiety, or depression, as these are an important part of your overall health.

✦ Have a record of your medical history. This should include past hospitalizations, surgeries, medical illnesses, immunizations, and test results from other doctors and specialists. Let your doctor know if your parents, siblings, or children had or have any serious medical conditions or diseases.

✦ Tell your doctor if you have any allergies or intolerances to foods or medications.

✦ Bring a list of all your medications with you. This should include herbal medicines, vitamins, and supplements that you buy over the counter, and those that other doctors prescribed for you. Let your physician know if you are having any side effects that you think might be caused by the medications.

✦ Let your doctor know if finances are a concern when discussing treatment. If money is tight, you might be able to use another, less expensive, generic medication that will work just as well.

Before you leave the office, make sure you have a clear sense of your current state of health and what screening tests you should have done. Ask your doctor if there are any lifestyle changes she recommends that could improve your health. And make sure you get the okay to engage in physical activities that will increase your heart rate, so you can move on to the next important step in your beauty/brain makeover.

Get a Second Opinion When:

✦ Your doctor dismisses your concerns.
✦ You are not satisfied with the care you are receiving.
✦ You're not getting better or therapies don't seem to be working.
✦ Your diagnosis is unclear or rare.
✦ Any nonstandard elective surgery is recommended.

TIP: If you need a second opinion, try a doctor at a facility that is different from the one where your doctor is affiliated. Physicians who know each other are often reluctant to contradict a colleague. You might also want to consider using a tertiary care or teaching hospital where cutting-edge therapies are being developed.

When a Sneeze Makes You Ill at Ease

I f you are like the millions of women who suffer from urinary incontinence, the simple act of sneezing will cause the involuntary release of urine. There are many causes of urinary incontinence, including stretching of pelvic floor muscles from childbirth, weight gain, deconditioning, menopause, and neurologic conditions. As part of my neurologic evaluation, I routinely ask women about bladder control. I often discover that women have not previously discussed bladder problems with their doctor because they are too embarrassed. Fortunately, most bladder control problems can be improved or cured, so let your doctor know if you have this problem and don't let incontinence "dampen" your social life.

Your Naked Brain

Did you ever wonder what your brain would look like if it were naked in front of a mirror? Would it look as fit as an Olympian athlete or out of shape and in desperate need of a makeover? The answer depends on your general health and lifestyle.

A female brain weighs about 2.5 pounds, which is less than 2 percent of our total body weight (based on the average weight of women being 164 pounds). It has the consistency of Brie cheese, and the area in between the furrows, called the gyri, should be plump with a rosy blush, indicating a healthy perfusion of blood, like that rosy-cheeked glow. An unhealthy brain, on the other hand, is shriveled and lackluster with a decidedly poor complexion.

If our mirror could magnify the tissue of a healthy brain just below the surface, we might see the outer layer (referred to as the "cortex" or as "gray matter") jam-packed with robust neurons (brain cells). The unhealthy brain, by contrast, would have fewer and more meager neurons with scattered remnants of brain cells that had died off. If we delved even deeper, we would see the "white matter," which are like wires that connect the cells forming its neural pathways and makes up 50 percent of our brain tissue. The white matter should be smooth, uniform, and glistening, while an unfit brain has blemishes—patchy areas of discoloration—and thinning pockmarked pathways.

If your brain is fit, the arteries would be supple, wide open, and free of debris to allow maximal blood flow. Arteries of a sluggish brain would be stiff and clogged with cholesterol-laden plaques that choke off the brain's supply of blood. Whatever the naked truth is about your brain, the good news is that you can improve your brain's appearance by changing your lifestyle to ensure that both your body and brain are hale, hearty, and gorgeous!

FOGGY BRAIN

Have you ever walked into a room and not been able to remember why you were there? Do you ever forget where you left your keys, or have the name of your high school math teacher stuck frustratingly on the tip of your tongue? Whether it's from work, stress, or lack of sleep, when our bodily systems are out of whack, the brain can no longer function at its best. The normal communication between our brain cells and activity within the brain gets altered or interrupted. This can manifest in a variety of "foggy brain" symptoms, including mental cloudiness, impaired memory, and a host of other neurologic problems.

There is no need to panic about these common memory lapses, and they do not necessarily mean you are losing your mind or sinking into a quicksand of senility. Taking care of your health, getting enough sleep, and the other tips in our brain makeover program will help relieve many of your foggy brain symptoms.

Still, as a neurologist, I have many patients and friends who ask me if they might be in the early stages of Alzheimer's disease. Whether it's a young patient seeing me for migraines or a friend who is in her later years, I am struck by how often I hear this concern. Patients referred to me specifically for memory problems typically enter my office in a panic—and understandably so. Losing control of our mental capabilities is one of our greatest fears because it means we are losing control over our lives.

One of the first things I tell concerned patients and friends is that there are countless treatable conditions that might be causing or contributing to their memory lapses, such as a vitamin deficiency or a hormonal imbalance. Again, many of the conditions that masquerade as dementia are reversible. I also can reassure my patients and friends, and you, that certain changes in brain function are simply a normal part of living longer. As we get older, the speed at which we process information slows down, and our memory may not be as strong as it was when we were younger. As frustrating as this can be, I encourage my friends and patients to appreciate those aspects of brain function that improve with age (yes, you read correctly—some things do get better!), such as our ability to make wise decisions.

Over time we develop a larger reservoir of knowledge to draw upon, allowing us to consider things more broadly and to see the whole picture better than someone who has not had as much experience. Our emotional circuits have less influence on our behavior and judgments, so we don't act as impulsively. We become more thoughtful. This is what we mean by wisdom, which confers that sense of peace, calm, and deep intelligence within. It is the gift and the beauty of the mature mind.

Whether I suspect patients are having memory problems due to an unhealthy lifestyle, a treatable medical condition, or early-onset Alzheimer's disease, my approach and prescription are the same. I take a thorough medical history, including symptoms, past health problems, and a review of their medical record. I ask what medications and supplements they are taking and review their family history. I also ask them about their lifestyle choices, including personal habits and social life.

Next I perform a physical and neurologic exam. If needed, I'll order additional testing, such as blood work or imaging studies (such as MRIs or CT scans). Then I'll review the results with my patients and make specific recommendations based on what I determine to be the underlying cause of their symptoms. Whatever the diagnosis turns out to be, whether it is Alzheimer's disease, depression masquerading as dementia, or simply sleep deprivation, we sit down and carefully go over the important steps they can take to ensure that their brain is functioning at its best. These are the same steps that I am sharing with you in this book.

Becky's Story

Becky had been looking forward to returning to work four months after the birth of her second child. As a journalist for a local paper, she enjoyed the mental stimulation of new assignments and the flexible hours. She became concerned when she started forgetting the details that, in the past, had been so easy for her to remember. Her writing took much longer and lacked some of the style and insight that it once possessed. She initially attributed her symptoms to Mommy Brain and the demands of juggling work and caring for two young children.

She tried taking better care of herself by going to bed earlier and eating nourishing meals, but she continued to have trouble focusing and started feeling exhausted and depressed. "I thought I was losing it," she confessed. Her husband and friends also noticed that something was terribly wrong. She had come to me for migraines in the past, so she decided to see me again. I immediately noticed that the usual sparkle in her eyes was missing. After hearing her story and performing a physical and neurologic exam, I had a hunch that she might be suffering from hypothyroidism. Thyroid dysfunction is especially common after childbirth, and Becky was exhibiting some of the classic symptoms.

A quick blood test confirmed my diagnosis. Within a few months of taking a prescription for thyroid medication, Becky's concentration and memory improved, her energy level returned, and her depression lifted. She was as good as ever and relieved that her mind was not in decline after all. So if your thinking is foggy, be sure to see your doctor.

What Is Dementia?

Dementia is the umbrella term for the loss of cognitive function, such as reasoning and memory, that is severe enough to interfere with daily life. There are many types of dementia, including Alzheimer's disease, a neurodegenerative disease that involves the loss or dying off of the brain cells over time. Other lesser-known neurodegenerative diseases that cause dementia include Lewy Body Dementia and Pick's Disease. Dementia can also be caused by a series of strokes, alcohol and drug abuse, or head trauma (either a single injury or multiple blows), as well as infections such as AIDS and Creutzfeldt-Jakob Disease.

According to a 2000 report from the World Health Organization (WHO), approximately 6 to 10 percent of the population sixty-five years and older in North America have dementia, with Alzheimer's accounting for two-thirds of those cases. Sadly there is no cure for Alzheimer's at this time. There are medications available that help treat the symptoms, but they have only a marginal benefit and do not prevent the progression of the disease. Yet another reason why we must do everything in our power to see to it that our brain stays healthy and fit for as long as possible!

BRAIN BEAUTY ESSENTIALS

There are two essential elements to brain health that can help us achieve a long-lasting, beautiful mind: The first involves going with the flow—blood flow, that is. Every cell in our body depends on a constant supply of blood to survive, which carries oxygen and nutrients to our cells and flushes out carbon dioxide and other waste products. As the Austrian poet Rainer Maria Rilke correctly observed, "All the soarings of my mind begin in my blood." But no other organ requires as much blood flow as the brain. Even though it makes up only 2 percent of our body, it uses a full 20 percent of the body's blood flow to meet its insatiable metabolic needs.

This is because neurons (brain cells) are the most highly specialized and vulnerable cells in the body and will die off in minutes without the proper blood flow. In contrast, fat cells are particularly hardy and can survive for hours without oxygen. It's one of nature's unfair pranks that makes it so hard to lose five pounds and so easy to lose brain cells! Maximizing blood flow to your brain is vital to keeping your mind beautifully fit.

Another important Brain Beauty Essential is avoiding "chronic inflammation." If you've ever sprained your ankle or burned your skin, you know how the affected areas become immediately inflamed. Inflammation is our body's natural healing response to injury, infection, allergy, or toxic exposure. But when our immune system doesn't turn itself off or is inappropriately triggered by unhealthy lifestyle choices and disease, the result is chronic inflammation.

Chronic inflammation is usually silent and difficult to diagnose. But it is believed to play a key role in the aging of the body and the brain. It leads to atherosclerosis (hardening of the arteries), which reduces blood flow and also interferes with normal cellular functions. Not surprisingly, stroke, poor cognitive function, and Alzheimer's disease have also been linked to chronic inflammation. Avoiding what I call the Brain Beauty Burglars will help keep your brain and your body beautiful.

BRAIN BEAUTY BURGLARS

There are numerous health conditions that can rob our brain of its enormous power and beauty. Fortunately many of them can be controlled or reversed by making the proper lifestyle changes that we recommend in your beauty/brain makeover. For starters, let's identify the culprits.

High Blood Pressure

High blood pressure damages the arteries that nourish the brain. Under pressure, arteries lose elasticity and the linings become rough and irritated, which causes plaque to develop. As the arteries eventually become clogged and narrow, the blood flow is decreased, which requires the heart to pump harder to do its job. This increases the pressure throughout the system. Hypertension (another name for high blood pressure) is one of the major risk factors for stroke, heart disease, and dementia. Studies show that if left untreated, hypertension can actually shrink your brain over time.

Remarkably, nearly one-third of people who have hypertension aren't aware they have it! And among those who are treated, less than half are successfully controlled, according to the American Heart Association. The reason for this scary statistic is that high blood pressure rarely has any symptoms, which allows it to sneak into your body and your brain unnoticed. Fortunately this Brain Beauty Burglar can be easily detected by a simple blood pressure check, and even small lifestyle changes, such as a healthful diet, exercise, and learning to "make over your mind" (see Step five) can prevent its entry. And if lifestyle changes don't do the trick, there is an arsenal of medicines that surely will, so there is no reason not to get a regular blood pressure check.

High Cholesterol

Unhealthy cholesterol levels cause plaque buildup and inflammation in the lining of blood vessels, resulting in decreased blood flow to the brain. High cholesterol levels have been linked to an increased risk of stroke and dementia. One study published in the *Archives of Neurology* found that, among female subjects, the higher LDL (bad cholesterol) and total cholesterol they had, the worse they did on cognitive testing.

Like hypertension, high cholesterol levels can slip under the radar as they stealthily begin to clog up arteries. A simple blood test readily spots this villain, which can be eliminated by following the Smart Diet (see Step six) and strategizing a plan of attack with your personal physician.

High Blood Sugar

Elevated blood sugar is another crafty scoundrel that wreaks havoc on your body from head to toe. It especially takes a toll on your brain. Diabetes is a chronic disease marked by high levels of glucose (sugar) in the blood. Type 2 diabetes (adult onset) is the most common form of diabetes. Prior to developing Type 2 diabetes, most people have "prediabetes," characterized by blood glucose levels that are higher than normal but not yet high enough to be diagnosed as diabetes.

Recent research has shown that long-term damage to the body seen in diabetics begins to occur during prediabetes. Diabetes damages blood vessels throughout the body, which increases the risk of heart attack and stroke. It is also the leading cause of blindness, kidney failure, and neuropathy (dysfunction of the peripheral nerves). Uncontrolled diabetes can also lead to thinning of the brain's cortex, and it increases the risk of Alzheimer's disease and other dementias.

Once again, making the appropriate lifestyle changes, including eating the Smart Diet, living dynamically through movement, and beautifying your brain rhythms by getting enough sleep can prevent diabetes or significantly improve blood sugar levels in those who have it. (See Steps four, six, and seven.) If needed, there are a variety of medications now available to combat this nasty brain beauty thief.

Obesity and Abdominal Fat

Obesity, particularly when fat is stored around the waist, is often the first invader who leaves the door open for the above three accomplices to make their entry. For years obesity has been a well-known risk factor for hypertension, high cholesterol, and diabetes, and consequently cardiovascular disease. Only recently, however, have scientists come to appreciate that obesity and abdominal girth also carry an increased risk for stroke and dementia.

In a groundbreaking study that spanned nearly three decades, Rachel Whitmer, Ph.D., found that people who were obese in middle age had a 74 percent increased risk of dementia than those of normal weight. She also discovered that, among those with normal weight in midlife, those who had the largest waists were twice as likely to get dementia as those with the smallest tummies. (Abdominal fat is thought to cause chronic inflammation throughout the body.)

I realize that the prospect of losing weight can be overwhelming. But I'm here to tell you that by taking charge of your brain you can learn to control your thoughts, your actions, and ultimately your weight. During your beauty/brain makeover, your mind will become clearer and stronger. But in order to improve your body you must first improve your mind. We will talk more about how to Make Over Your Mind in Step five.

Smoking

Nearly all smokers already know that it's a difficult addiction and have probably tried just about everything to snuff it out. Giving up cigarettes is arguably the single most important action you must take if you are truly serious about keeping your body and brain healthy. Smoking is a well-known risk factor for vascular disease, heart disease, stroke, lung cancer, and multiple other cancers as well as countless other physical ailments. Most recently smoking has also been linked to an increased risk for dementia and Alzheimer's disease. It decreases blood flow to the brain, and the tobacco toxins promote inflammation.

So please don't give up just because you've failed to quit in the past. Talk to your doctor about nicotine replacement therapies and other medications. As with every other step in your makeover, there's no reason why you should go it alone, so look for local smoking cessation groups in your area or ask your Beautiful Brain Buddy to be your "sponsor" and call her whenever you feel the urge to light up.

STROKE—THE MOST NOTORIOUS BRAIN BEAUTY THIEF

The Brain Beauty Burglars mentioned above compromise blood flow to the brain and/or promote inflammation, all of which can pave the way for the most notorious brain beauty thief of all—stroke. A stroke occurs when blood flow to part of the brain is interrupted, and the lack of oxygen and nutrients causes brain cells to die. There are various ways that this can happen. Blocked arteries are the most common cause of stroke. Arteries can gradually get blocked over time or become suddenly blocked by a blood clot. Blood clots arise from inflamed arterial plaques and from an unhealthy heart. When these blood clots break off and travel in the bloodstream to the brain, they become lodged in an artery. When this happens, the area of brain supplied by that artery will die.

Another cause of stroke is a ruptured blood vessel in the brain. This causes a "cerebral hemorrhage" or bleeding within the brain. Uncontrolled hypertension is the most common cause of a cerebral hemorrhage. Abnormalities in cerebral blood vessels, including aneurysms (an abnormal ballooning out of the vessel wall) and arteriovenous malformations or AVM (an abnormal collection of blood vessels), can also cause bleeding in the brain.

The hallmark of a ruptured aneurysm or AVM is a severe headache that comes on suddenly and reaches its maximum intensity in seconds. Patients often describe this abrupt onset headache as similar to being "hit in the head with a bat." The headache is sometimes accompanied by a stiff neck due to blood tracking around the brain and down the spinal cord. Needless to say, a stroke and bleeding in the brain are neurologic emergencies. Brain cells are dying and immediate medical attention is required.

The symptoms of stroke depend on what part of the brain is deprived of blood flow. If a motor pathway is affected, for example, the ability to move will be impaired. If language areas are deprived of blood flow, the person may have trouble understanding what people are saying, appear confused, or have difficulty speaking. In some cases, a person might not even be aware that she is having a stroke because the part of the brain that perceives changes in the body is affected.

Stroke symptoms usually develop suddenly and without warning, or they may occur on and off for the first day or two. Sometimes symptoms may completely disappear within a few minutes. This can happen when a blood clot initially lodged in an artery breaks up on its own and blood flow is resumed. This is called a "TIA" (transient ischemic attack) or "stroke warning." The risk of having a full-blown stroke is very high after a TIA. For this reason, you must call 911 immediately if you have any of the symptoms of a stroke warning, even if the symptoms disappear completely. And remember, the best way to prevent stroke is to avoid the Brain Beauty Burglars listed above.

"Give Me 5!"

Research presented at the 2009 International Stroke Conference showed that only 37 percent of people surveyed knew the five warning signs of stroke that warranted an immediate 911 call. Because this is such a huge concern within the medical community, the American Academy of Neurology, the American College of Emergency Physicians, and the American Stroke Association launched the "Give Me 5! for Stroke" campaign to raise stroke awareness.

The Give Me 5! campaign reminds us to consider a series of "Walk, Talk, Reach, See, Feel" questions if you are with someone who might be having a stroke. As a neurologist, it is heartbreaking for me to see patients living with a neurologic disability that could have been prevented had they only known the symptoms of stroke. To that end, I hope you will remember the following five symptoms and Give Me 5!

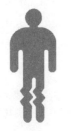

1. **WALK**
    ✦ Is their balance off?
    ✦ Are they dragging one leg?
    ✦ Are they veering off to one side?

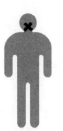

2. **TALK**

+ Is their speech slurred?
+ Are they using the appropriate words? (Do their words make sense?)
+ Does one side of their mouth droop down?

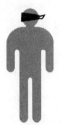

3. **REACH**

+ Is one side weak or numb?
+ Ask the person to raise both their arms up together. Does one arm begin to fall down?
+ Ask the person to squeeze your fingers with each hand. Is one hand weaker than the other?

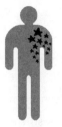

4. **SEE**

+ Is their vision all or partly lost?
+ Is their vision clear?
+ Does the person see double?

5. **FEEL**

+ Do they have a severe headache that peaked in severity within seconds?
+ Do they normally have headaches? If so, is this headache any different from their usual headache?
+ Does this feel like the worst headache of their life?

When to Call 911

Having a stroke means brain cells are dying, so getting to a hospital as quickly as possible gives you or the victim the best chance of recovery. Although the risk of stroke does increase with age, it is important to know that strokes can occur at any age, even in children! If a stroke is due to a blocked artery, Tissue Plasminogen Activator (tPA) can be given to break up the clot and restore blood flow. This medicine must be given within the first three hours after the onset of stroke symptoms. Studies show it can increase the risk of bleeding complications if given after three hours, which could worsen the outcome. However, when given promptly, tPA can reverse or reduce the symptoms of stroke and decrease permanent disability. This is why it is so important to get to the hospital ASAP. Unfortunately, many people do not arrive at the hospital within this three-hour window and therefore miss out on this effective treatment. And even when tPA cannot be administered, there are other measures that doctors can take to limit the disability and aftereffects of stroke. So the bottom line is: If you think you or a loved one is having a stroke, call 911 immediately.

What You Should Know about Stroke in Women

Did you know that twice as many women die of stroke as breast cancer every year and that stroke is the third leading cause of death in women after heart disease and cancer? Chronic lung disease is fourth, and Alzheimer's is fifth. Despite these sobering statistics, most women worry much more about their risk of getting breast cancer. While we can live without our breasts, we cannot live without our brain!

Women are also more likely than men to have nontraditional stroke symptoms. Although women are most likely to experience the Give Me 5! stroke symptoms listed above, it's important to be aware of the lesser-known symptoms of stroke in women. According to a study in the *Annals of Emergency Medicine*, the most common nontraditional symptoms for women are decreased alertness, unconsciousness, and sudden pain—typically on one side of the body. Other less common nontraditional stroke symptoms include sudden-onset hiccups, nausea, shortness of breath, chest pain, and palpitations.

Women are also less likely to have the traditional symptoms of a heart attack. Although chest pain or discomfort is the most common heart attack symptom for women, some present with pain in the neck, jaw, shoulder, or abdomen. Others may not have any pain but instead experience shortness of breath, nausea or vomiting, sweating, lightheadedness, dizziness, or unusual fatigue. Did you notice the overlap of atypical symptoms for women with stroke and heart attack? In addition to using the Give Me 5! checklist, if you are experiencing any of the symptoms listed above, call 911 ASAP.

Female Hormones and Stroke

Female hormones, including birth control pills and hormone replacement therapy (HRT), have been found to increase the risk of stroke among women. The risk of stroke also increases during pregnancy, a time when our hormonal levels are elevated. In younger women who do not have other stroke risk factors, such as smoking, birth control pills are generally considered safe. In addition to stroke, the 2002 Women's Health Initiative Study also found a rise in heart disease and breast cancer among women taking HRT. Since then, postmenopausal women have been advised to use HRT under limited circumstances and only for the shortest period of time possible.

Migraines and Stroke

Migraine headaches, which women get more often than men, are also linked to female hormones. Migraines commonly start in the teenage years when women begin to menstruate. They tend to be more frequent and severe around the time of menstruation, when hormonal levels fluctuate dramatically. They also frequently flare up during perimenopause, the years leading up to menopause.

Some women experience neurologic symptoms with their migraines called "auras," which typically last between ten and twenty minutes and include seeing flashing lights, zigzag lines, and blind spots. Auras can also cause numbness, tingling, or speech problems. Not surprisingly, many women seek medical attention with their first migraine aura and justifiably so, since the symptoms resemble those of a TIA or stroke warning. In fact, medical tests such as a brain MRI are often done to ascertain the diagnosis.

Having migraine headaches slightly increases one's chances of having a stroke, especially for migraine with aura. The overall risk, however, is still extremely low. Keep in mind that migraines are very common (I have them myself), but when combined with other factors such as birth control pills, this risk increases. If you are taking birth control pills and have migraine with aura, you should talk to your doctor about using other forms of birth control. Anyone who suffers from migraine should also ask their doctor about the many effective medications that are available to both prevent and stop migraine headaches.

Susan's Story

Susan, a sixty-three-year-old schoolteacher who lives alone, arrived home after a long day at work. As she tried to unlock the door, the keys repeatedly fell out of her right hand. She thought this was peculiar, but she managed to compensate by turning the key with her left hand and proceeded to put the incident behind her.

Later that evening, Susan noticed that she was having difficulty holding the newspaper that she was reading. "I didn't have the strength to hold my right hand up," she later told me. "I wondered if I might be having a stroke. But within five minutes my hand seemed perfectly fine, so I decided not to worry about it and went to bed."

When she awoke the next morning, she was paralyzed on her right side. She managed to dial 911 but, unfortunately, it was too late to give her the clot-busting tPA that might have reversed her symptoms. Had she heeded the warning signs the night before and gone to the hospital earlier, her doctors would likely have prevented the stroke from occurring in the first place.

KNOW YOUR NUMBERS

Now that I've told you what to look out for in order to keep your body and brain in tip-top condition, I want to help you decipher what all those confusing test numbers mean. And while we're at it, I'll show you how to determine your ideal body mass index (BMI) by using the following chart. Please don't get discouraged if your numbers aren't where they should be right now. Think of them as goals that you are setting for yourself and give yourself time to follow the program and get to where you want to be. These tests are the compasses we doctors use to guide our patients toward the right treatment and, in this case, to help you jump-start (or complete) your beauty/brain makeover.

Blood Pressure

Blood pressure is measured by two numbers. The top number (systolic pressure) is the highest pressure inside your arteries, measured at the moment when your heart contracts. The bottom number (diastolic pressure) is the lowest pressure in your arteries, measured while your heart is relaxing in between beats. Ideally, your blood pressure should be under 120/80. However this will vary, depending on your age and other medical conditions. Discuss with your doctor what the best blood pressure is for you.

BMI (Body Mass Index)

Your BMI, which is based on your weight and height, predicts your risk for developing many chronic diseases, including diabetes, heart and vascular disease, high blood pressure, liver disease, osteoarthritis, sleep disorders, and cancer. The risk of developing these chronic diseases increases significantly in the "overweight" range of BMI 25–29 and even more notably in the "obese" range over 30. A BMI in the obese range can also increase your risk of stroke and dementia.

Use the following chart to determine your BMI category. Find your height in the first column, then move across that row to your approximate weight range. The numbers at the bottom of the column indicate your BMI range and category. It is best to be in the normal range of 19–24; but if you're not there yet, stick with the program, and you'll get there eventually.

BODY MASS INDEX

HEIGHT	BODY WEIGHT IN POUNDS				
4'10"	91–115	119–138	143–162	167–186	191+
4'11"	94–119	124–143	148–168	173–193	198+
5'0"	97–123	128–148	153–174	179–199	204+
5'1"	100–127	132–153	158–180	185–206	211+
5'2"	104–131	136–158	164–186	191–213	218+
5'3"	107–135	141–163	169–191	197–220	225+
5'4"	110–140	145–169	174–197	204–227	232+
5'5"	114–144	150–174	180–204	210–234	240+
5'6"	118–148	155–179	186–210	216–241	247+
5'7"	121–153	159–185	191–217	223–249	255+
5'8"	125–158	164–190	197–223	230–256	262+
5'9"	128–162	169–196	203–230	236–263	270+
5'10"	132–167	174–202	209–236	243–271	278+
5'11"	136–172	179–208	215–243	250–279	286+
6'0"	140–177	184–213	221–250	258–287	294+
6'1"	144–182	189–219	227–257	265–295	302+
6'2"	148–186	194–225	233–264	272–303	311+
6'3"	152–192	200–232	240–272	279–311	319+
6'4"	156–197	205–238	246–279	287–320	328+
BMI	19–24	25–29	30–34	35–39	40+
	NORMAL	OVER-WEIGHT	CLASS I OBESITY	CLASS II OBESITY	CLASS III OBESITY

Waist Circumference

Take a tape measure and put one end on your belly button and wrap it around your waist. Ideally your girth should measure less than half your height. This means, if you are five foot four (sixty-four inches), for example, the average female height, your waist should be less than thirty-two inches. If your waist is more than half your height, that indicates excessive abdominal fat, which is linked to diabetes, vascular disease, heart disease, stroke, and dementia.

Keep in mind that most women don't have Barbie Doll waists, so don't despair if you are shaped more like an apple than a pear. Genetics play a big part in how our bodies look, so all we can do is the best we can with what we've got. We're striving for health and fitness, not heavenly bodies! That said, I have suggestions later on for what kinds of food you should eat and exercises you can do to shrink your waistline.

FASTING LIPID PANEL

A fasting lipid panel measures the fats in the blood. It includes your total cholesterol, your "good" cholesterol (high-density lipoprotein/HDL), your "bad" cholesterol (low-density lipoprotein/LDL), and your triglycerides. They are all important, and you need to know the results. There's a lot of confusion between HDL, the good cholesterol that keeps arteries healthy, and LDL, the bad cholesterol that clogs them up. An easy way to remember which should be high and which should be low is in the name. For HDL (high-density lipoprotein) *high* levels are better, while for LDL (low-density lipoprotein) *low* levels are desirable.

Here's what you should aim for:

+ **Total Cholesterol**
  Less than 200 milligrams (good)
  201–240 mg/dL (borderline)
  Greater than 240 mg/dL (high)

+ **HDL (Good Cholesterol); higher is better**
  Greater than 60 milligrams (good)
  40–59 mg/dL (acceptable)
  Less than 40 mg/dL (low)

+ **LDL (Bad Cholesterol); lower is better**
  Less than 100 milligrams (good)
  100–129 mg/dL or less (acceptable)
  130–159 (borderline high)
  Greater than 160 mg/dL (high)

+ **Triglycerides**
  Less than 150 mg/dL (good)
  150–199 mg/dL (borderline high)
  Greater than 200 mg/dL (high)

The guidelines above only apply to those without cardiovascular risk factors such as hypertension, diabetes, or smoking. As you probably know, interpreting lipid panels can be complicated. This is just one reason why it is important to have a good relationship with your doctor. Ask your doctor what is best for you.

Fasting Blood Sugar

A healthy level is under 100. A fasting blood sugar in the range of 100 to 125 indicates prediabetes, while a level higher than 126 indicates diabetes. In most cases, proper diet and exercise, which we will talk about later, can lower blood sugar levels to the normal range. Often losing as little as five to ten pounds and being more active can make a significant difference.

Other Tests

These are additional tests that your doctor may recommend based on your age, symptoms, and risk factors.

Thyroid function: An imbalance of thyroid hormones wreaks havoc in both the brain and body. Low levels can cause mental fogginess, fatigue, excessive sleep, depression, weight gain, and hair loss. High levels can cause nervousness, decreased concentration, tremor, heat intolerance, palpitations, and weight loss. This hormone is easily repleted with medication if low, and there is excellent treatment for high levels as well.

Vitamin B12 level: This vitamin is important for maintaining healthy nerve cells and red blood cells. B12 deficiency can be caused by inadequate dietary intake or an inability to absorb B12 in the gut. B12 deficiency can cause anemia in addition to a host of neurologic symptoms, including mental confusion, mood change, and sensory disturbances. Most cases of B12 deficiency can be treated with oral supplements. For those who are unable to absorb B12, a monthly injection will do the trick.

Vitamin D level: This important vitamin is obtained from diet as well as from sunshine. Its role in maintaining healthy bones has been known for years. More recently, vitamin D deficiency has been linked to cognitive impairment, stroke, heart disease, muscle weakness, diabetes, obesity, depression, and multiple sclerosis. If you live in northern latitudes, avoid sun exposure, or have dark skin, or if you take certain medications or have kidney disease, you have an increased risk of vitamin D deficiency. Like B12 deficiency, this can usually be treated with over-the-counter supplements. Occasionally prescription-strength vitamin D is needed.

I hope you have a better understanding of how your body affects your brain and why taking good care of it will help you to live a longer, healthier, and more radiant life. I also hope you won't hesitate to ask your doctor (or find one whom you trust to ask) about anything concerning your health, no matter how insignificant, embarrassing, or scary it might seem. Knowledge is power, and it can change your life and your brain, which is exactly what this program is all about!

GET READY TO GLOW

Now that you understand how caring for your body helps you take care of your mind, it's time to engage in what I call Dynamic Living. Dynamic Living involves increasing the pace of your heart, rather than simply going through the paces. Once you've gotten your doctor's permission to increase your pulse to your heart's—and brain's—delight, you can hit the ground running (or spinning, or dancing, or jumping). You guessed it, the next step in your beauty/brain makeover is to get your face glowing and your blood flowing. The following step will explain what neurologists already know—the more you move and the more physically active you are, the more limber your brain will be and the better you will look and feel throughout your lifetime!

Go for the Glow!

Never put an age limit on your dreams.

—Dara Torres, Olympic silver
medalist at age forty-one

To say that exercise is good for your health is a no-brainer. But as we do with the warning on cigarette packs, many of us choose to ignore what is common knowledge and sound advice. Some people, women especially, seem either to hate the idea of exercise or feel they don't have time between work, family, and other obligations. If any of this is true for you, this step in your makeover is one of the most important ones you will take. I promise not to preach or wag a guilt-provoking finger, but I will give you scientifically proven reasons why movement not only is good for your body but can also turn back the biological clock for your brain!

For starters, when we move our body and our blood starts pumping, our cheeks flush, our brow becomes damp, and our faces glow. That "glow" is not just superficial—your brain is also enjoying and reaping the benefits of rejuvenating blood flow. This increased blood flow physically alters the brain, bathing it in a cascade of growth factors that promote the birth of new brain cells and create stronger neural connections.

In other words, the physical changes that take place in your brain when you are active allow it to work better and become more resilient to disease. Dr. John Ratey, a Harvard psychiatrist, refers to these growth factors released during exercise as "Miracle-Gro" for the brain. Moving your body literally transforms your brain—making it stronger, healthier, and ultimately more vibrant. It enhances concentration, learning, and memory; it uplifts our mood; and it relieves anxiety. And perhaps most important, research shows that physical activity helps stave off dementia as we age.

Now let's talk about how regular exercise changes the way we look. It rejuvenates the skin by improving blood flow, which makes skin appear smooth and supple. Physical activity makes us leaner by burning fat, regulates our appetite, tones our muscles, strengthens our bones, and improves our posture and balance. When we are active, the blood that surges throughout our body also flows into our sexual organs, which heightens our libido and sexual responsiveness. And when we feel better about the way we look, we are more confident in and out of bed. (Exercise also helps us sleep better, which we will talk more about in Step seven.) Exercise not only makes you look younger, but you will also actually *test* younger by a variety of physiologic measures. In short, exercise is the greatest beauty/brain prescription around, so why not go for that radiant healthy glow through what I call Dynamic Living?

Dynamic Living is anything that quickens your pulse and gets your blood pumping. And it doesn't have to involve getting on a treadmill or joining a gym. Once again, I will ask you to indulge in the new, only this time we will explore new ways to incorporate more activity into your life. Whether you're a Newbie, for whom exercise has been getting in and out of your car; a Gonnabe, who would love to be fit but doesn't know how to fit it into her schedule; or a Trainiac, who like me can't get enough of those feel-good endorphins, there's a Dynamic Living program for you. I will also show how physical activity can be a social activity, and, like everything else in this book, it is better when you join up with a buddy or a group of friends. To that end, I'm going to substitute the term "playout" for "workout" because exercise shouldn't be work—it should be fun!

My husband jokingly calls exercise my "psychotherapy," and he's right, but it goes far beyond that: Exercise rejuvenates my mind *and* my spirit. For me, it's a celebration of health. It keeps my mood sunny, clears my mind, and helps me deal with the pain and suffering that I see every day. One of the things I appreciate about practicing medicine is the poignant reminder that we can all lose our health in a heartbeat. For me, physical activity is a way to celebrate the gift of living and being able to breathe deeply and move my body. Whether I'm moving in time with other women in dance class, swooshing down a wintry slope, or running along the streets of my hometown, exercise is a spiritual act that fills my heart with gratitude.

EXERCISE HELPS US THINK

Did you know that just a single session of aerobic exercise can improve our mental processes? This was what Charles Hillman, Ph.D., concluded in his study at the University of Illinois at Urbana-Champaign, where he recruited twenty college-aged men and women to work out at a moderate intensity on a treadmill for thirty minutes on multiple occasions. At one session, the participants were asked to take a cognitive test before they exercised; at another, they took the test afterward. When they worked out on the treadmill before the test, they showed improved reaction time and memory. Hillman also tested the participants after non-aerobic resistance exercise. There was no improvement. Only those who performed aerobic exercise before the test showed better concertration and recall. According to Hillman, this could mean that people who exercise are able to multitask at a greater speed while making more accurate decisions.

Again and again, research has shown that moving your body literally makes your brain stronger, healthier, and ultimately more vibrant. In another recent study of only women published in *Neurobiology of Aging*, those subjects who were the most physically fit were found to have better blood flow to their brain and to perform better on tests of memory and reasoning than women who were less fit.

GET A MOOD-LIFT

In addition to enhancing concentration, learning, and memory, exercise also improves our mood and helps relieve anxiety. Studies show that people who exercise regularly benefit from a boost in mood and lower rates of depression and anxiety. In fact exercise can be as effective as antidepressants at treating mild to moderate depression without the side effect of weight gain, which is common for many mood-enhancing medications. The increased blood flow of exercise causes the release of feel-good neurotransmitters, including endorphins that trigger positive feelings in the short term. According to one recent study by the American College of Sports Medicine, cardio activity can elevate your mood for up to twelve hours. Plus the birth of new neurons that occurs with regular exercise is believed to play a central role in keeping spirits high in the long run.

Research also shows that exercise gives you more self-confidence by enhancing your body image and body satisfaction. Improving your physical strength and stamina is empowering because it gives you a sense of control over your body, your mind, and your life.

These are just some of the gifts of Dynamic Living, so whatever your age or current lifestyle, today is the day to go for the glow. If you are already active, find new ways to take it up a notch so you will reap even more brain and beauty benefits!

YOUR BRAIN'S FOUNTAIN OF YOUTH

As studies clearly prove, engaging in physical activity that increases your heart rate and builds stamina is like bathing your brain in a fountain of youth. How do all these beautifying changes take place in the brain when we move? Aerobic activity generates a compound called "brain-derived neurotrophic factor" (BDNF), which enhances "synaptic plasticity," or the ability of neurons to talk to one another. As we discussed in the first step, in order to learn something new, our brain has to make new connections, or synapses. When learning is reinforced, these connections become stronger. But as we get older, our synaptic connections decrease in both number and potency. Through the release of BDNF and other nerve growth factors, we can improve our ability to make new connections and to learn. BDNF not only promotes the birth of new neurons, it also supports the survival of *existing* neurons.

Remember the Brain Beauty Essentials we talked about in the last step? Activities that increase your heart rate maximize that very important blood flow. But the effect of cardio reaches far beyond lipid profiles and blood pressure readings—physical activity boosts our immune function, decreases inflammation, and encourages the growth of new blood vessels in both the brain and the body. It protects our brain from those Brain Beauty Burglars by promoting weight loss and increasing our good cholesterol while lowering our blood pressure, bad cholesterol, and blood sugar. Aerobic activity will make your brain more beautiful and decrease your risk of stroke and dementia. This brain beauty ritual is far too amazing to miss out on!

The Younger Your Cells, the Younger You Look

Wrinkles aren't the only ways we show the signs of aging. In fact, they are just a reflection of what is happening inside our cells. Aging begins at the cellular level, and our cells' chromosomes reveal the toll that life can take on our bodies. Studies have shown that psychological stress actually ages our cells by wearing down the ends of our chromosomes, called "telomeres."

Telomeres look like the tips of shoelaces, and they prevent our chromosomes from becoming unraveled or frayed. When they become worn by wear and tear, the length of our telomeres shrinks, which is a telltale sign of cellular aging. Every time a cell divides, its telomeres shorten. And when they become too short, the cell can no longer divide and will eventually die. But how quickly our telomeres shorten depends on how well we care for our body. Tim Spector, a professor at King's College, London, compared the telomere length of more than a thousand pairs of twins. Those who were more physically active had longer telomeres—in essence, younger-looking cells—compared to their twin siblings who were more sedentary.

In other words, genetics doesn't tell the whole story. The amount of exercise we get has a huge impact on how fast we age. Exercise makes your individual cells more youthful, which in turn makes you look younger from the inside out.

My Story

When I was in college, the aerobics movement was just getting started, and I taught an aerobics dance class on campus. It was a great way to earn money on the side, but more important, I learned about resilience and the transformative power of movement. There were days I would show up feeling tired or stressed about an upcoming exam and the last thing I felt like doing was teaching a class. But once I put the music on and looked at all of these wonderful women who had paid money to take my class, I felt obligated to make the experience worth their time and money. Wanting them to have fun, I forced an enthusiastic smile and turned up the energy. To my surprise, once I became absorbed by the movement, my smile and enthusiasm became genuine. (Remember when we talked about how faking a smile can actually make you feel happier?) By the end of the class, I felt exuberant, fulfilled, mentally clear, and ready to hit the books.

By repeating this experiment many times, I made an important discovery: Movement could transform my mind and body. I became stronger both physically and mentally, and experienced a new sense of inner happiness and confidence. My grades got better, and it improved every aspect of my life—it still does. It is my fervent wish that if you haven't started exercising yet, you will begin today, and if you already experience the joy of movement that you will keep on going!

Exercise Your Willpower

As you begin your Dynamic Living program, I want you to start using your strength of mind to help strengthen your body. Muscles get stronger by resisting the power of weights. Inner strength is achieved by overcoming inner resistance. We will focus on this in the next step as you "make over your mind," but for now, try the suggestions below to start fortifying your willpower:

✦ You get up in the morning and the bed is unmade. You don't want to take the time to straighten the covers, and besides, you tell yourself that you'll only mess them up again when you go to bed at night. Don't give in to the little voice that says, "Do it later." Suck it up and make your bed while you are thinking about it.

✦ You come home after a long, tiring day at work. You need to wash your hair, but you really want to relax and watch TV. Resist the temptation to crease the couch and instead beeline for the shower first.

✦ You continually say you are going to exercise but you never follow through on your promise. Before you go to bed tonight, go for a ten-minute walk or run, or lift weights. Resist the temptation to pull a Scarlett O'Hara and say, "I'll think about that tomorrow."

✦ You take the bus to work each day and always hope to get a seat for your commute. Instead try standing or giving up your seat to someone else for one week.

✦ You learn some interesting gossip about a co-worker and you're dying to tell another workmate. See how long you can go without uttering a word to anyone.

✦ You always have a bagel and cream cheese for breakfast in the morning. Try having a slice of whole grain toast and natural peanut butter instead.

✦ Your spouse leaves the dishes in the sink unwashed, despite your having asked him countless times to rinse them off or put them in the dishwasher. You want to lash out at him but instead you say, "I'll take care of your dishes today," and decide to let it go.

✦ You catch a glimpse of yourself in the mirror and are disgusted by that roll of flab around your belly. Your thoughts start drifting about how awful you look and how lazy you are. Stop the negative thoughts immediately and replace them with: "I'm going to start my Dynamic Living program today!"

DYNAMIC LIVING FOR NEWBIES

Now that you know what Dynamic Living can do for your brain, health, and longevity, the trick is finding an activity that you can start and stick with. One of the biggest hurdles Newbies face is the fear of looking foolish or feeling uncomfortable in their own body. Many women have negative body images because they compare themselves to Photoshopped or cosmetically altered images of models and celebrities.

Other times we opt out of physical activities because we feel we're not good enough, or we are simply overwhelmed by the prospect of getting in shape. Perhaps you've tried to be active in the past and have given it up. Take a moment to consider what's holding you back and preventing you from reaping the benefits of exercise.

As a neurologist, I can tell you that negative thoughts have a way of becoming reinforced and deeply embedded over time. The beauty of the brain, however, is that it's plastic and constantly changing. By replacing negative thoughts about exercise with positive ones you can weaken the old negative neural pathways and forge new positive ones in your brain.

When women tell me "I'm such a klutz" or "I hate to exercise," I tell them it's never too late to retrain your brain and start thinking differently. I ask them to replace those thoughts with positive affirmations such as "My body is beautiful and graceful" or "I breathe in joy with every step." Perhaps you never had a positive exercise experience. If the only exercise you've every tried was walking on a treadmill or running circles around a track, then you've yet to experience the variety that makes up Dynamic Living. When I talk to Trainiacs, I find that, like me, they were fortunate to find an activity or sport that they are passionate about.

You must start by changing the way you define physical activity. Don't like going to a gym and mingling among all the heavenly bodies? Gather some women of substance, ones who understand what it's like to live large, and get up and get out as a group. There is strength in numbers, and you will see how quickly you will all build up your own strength and self-confidence. The following strategies have inspired me and my patients to get moving.

Rediscover the Joy in Movement

Throughout this book, I talk about how passion is a powerful motivator—so why not pursue a physical passion? Is there a sport or activity that you enjoyed when you were younger but haven't done in years? Maybe you used to swim, hike, ice-skate, or jump on a trampoline. Did you play volleyball or soccer when you were in school? Mothers already know that kids are constantly on the move: hopping, skipping, and running—reveling in the sheer joy of being alive! Observe children at play and imagine feeling that breathless excitement again. Let your imagination wander and come up with some fun, new activities to pursue.

When was the last time you had fun moving? (Chances are it wasn't while doing calisthenics!) Perhaps memories of dancing at a friend's wedding, playing Frisbee on the beach, or skiing down a white powdery mountain bring back that feeling of being and moving in the moment. These are clues to what type of activities you need to bring into your life. Be creative and explore the possibilities.

Start a Walking Group

As I said earlier, physical activity can be a social activity, so gather up your friends and start a regular walking group. Making your daily constitutionals a group activity is guaranteed to prevent exercise from being a chore and a bore. Jane Brody, the *New York Times* personal health columnist, who is nearly seventy, wrote the following about her cherished daily walks with friends.

> Shortly after 6 the other morning, a stunning full moon hugging the horizon enhanced our walk around our local park, and I remarked, "Look what the stay-a-beds are missing." . . . Note that I said "we." Two to five of us walk for an hour every morning. We chat about our days, share our thoughts and problems, seek and offer advice, bolster sagging spirits, provide logistical support, alert one another to coming cultural events, discuss

the news, books, articles and what-have-you. No matter how awful I may feel when I get up in the morning, I always feel better after that walk.

To improve endurance, Newbies can try walking for ten seconds at a faster clip; then let the body recover before trying to speed it up again. You can increase your heart rate by "speed walking," which is picking up your pace while exaggerating your arm movements so they swing higher than normal. These "intervals," which I will discuss more later in this step, can be incorporated into almost any activity, whether you're walking to the bus stop, cruising through a shopping mall, or taking a flight of stairs. Pushing a stroller, wearing ankle weights, or carrying hand weights will increase your endurance and heart rate. You and the group can also improve your stamina by walking a little bit farther every day, week, month—depending on your fitness level and allotted time.

If you're the competitive type, challenge your friends to a walkoff. Get a pedometer that counts the number of steps you take and wear it for a day. The one with the most steps takes the others out for a nonfat frozen yogurt with fruit on top.

So You Think You Can Dance?

Sign up for two-stepping, ballroom, hip-hop, or folk dancing lessons with friends or a significant other. If you have two left feet, going with a pal will make it easier to laugh when you step on each other's toes. Go clubbing to practice your moves and make a fun night of it. Watch the dance contests on TV for inspiration, or get tickets to see a ballroom competition. (Remember the "mirror neurons" we talked about in Step two?) To find a contest near you, go to www.dance-forums.com/competitions/.

Check out local dance studios for beginner classes in tap, jazz, hip-hop, modern, or ballet. The beauty of taking classes as an adult is that you get to choose your instructor. Finding the right teacher makes all the difference in the world. It's worth shopping around for someone who will motivate you and make the class fun, and many studios will let you watch a class before signing up. Most instructors will teach a new routine every few weeks. Learning to move differently and memorizing new dances are fun ways to challenge your mind and will double the brain benefits. It doesn't matter what kind of dance you are doing as long as you are having fun shaking your booty!

Gotta Dance
(Who Says You Can't Hip-Hop at Eighty?)

The 2008 award-winning documentary *Gotta Dance* proved, as its press release trumpeted, "that age doesn't matter . . . unless you are a cheese." The movie, directed by Dori Berinstein, chronicled the debut of the New Jersey Nets' first-ever senior hip-hop dance team, The NJ NETSationals. The group of twelve women and one man made headlines after being chosen as cheerleaders in an *American Idol*–like audition. This delightful film, which is available on DVD, shows why age is a state of mind and how these inspirational people transformed their lives by learning dance steps and wowing the fans with their dare-to-break-a-hip–hop moves.

As Berinstein explains, "I wanted to make this film to celebrate age and to inspire and challenge present and future AARP members to embrace life—to get out there and take on something they always dreamed of doing." The members of the team include:

Peggy, 74: A former Miss Subways and prize-winning "jitter bugger."

Deanna, 65: Deanna played hooky from work to try out. She was caught by her boss when he saw her audition for the Nets dance team on the *Nightly News*.

Betty/Betsy, 64: Kindergarten teacher by day, hip-hop groupie by night.

Marge, 83: Marge's granddaughter Marla is a Nets Dancer and her new coach.

Fanny, 81: This line-dancing regular became a celebrity after her Filipino community saw her strut her stuff at the arena.

Willa, 74: A great-great grandmother who sports a new hairstyle every week. Willa says she's been fifty for twenty-four years.

Audrey, 60: Audrey was horrified when she turned sixty and lied to everyone about her age. Now she wears her age proudly on her jersey in front of an arena of cheering fans.

Get Inspired by Helping Others

If you are the altruistic type, you might find the inspiration to move by helping others. From shopping for a housebound neighbor and preparing dinner at a local shelter to helping a stressed-out mom by taking her children to the park, there are countless ways to weave more activity into your day while doing a good deed at the same time. Participate in the local park or beach cleanup, join the neighborhood gardening association, sign up for a charity walk, or become a Big Sister to an underprivileged child. All these activities will rejuvenate your body as well as your soul.

MENTAL PUSH-UPS FOR NEWBIES

Need a little motivation to keep you on track? I realize it's not easy to start something new, and it's even harder to see it through. So if you just started a new activity, please don't give up now! If you've yet to hear the starter gun, then get into a crouch position instead of couch position and practice doing the following mental push-ups:

✦ **Set achievable goals so you can see a tangible result.** Don't set the bar too high at first—for example, "I'm going to walk five miles this week." Aim for a "moderate" challenge instead. When something is too easy, we're apt to get bored, and if it is too hard we become discouraged and give up. So be kind to yourself and remember—finish lines can always be moved and bars can always be lifted.

✦ **Listen to your body.** There will be days when you need to take it easy on yourself. As Woody Allen said, "Eighty percent of success is showing up." So if you're feeling under the weather, shorten your workout, decrease the intensity, or just try again another day.

✦ **Find a cheering squad.** I've said it before, but I can't say it enough: Exercising with others will boost your motivation to a new level. If you take a class, get to know the teacher and the other participants. Try to seek out a teacher with a following, which means that the instructor has something special to offer. Parents want their children to have the best teachers, why not do this for yourself? Find a class with a magical atmosphere— they are out there. Or join a spirited softball, Ultimate Frisbee, or volleyball team. You will find that the motivation and support is wildly infectious. Remember how we talked in Step two about how emotions can be contagious? Think about the last time you went to a sporting event and sat among other fans in the bleachers. Rooting for one another will boost the fun as well as everyone's performance. And don't forget to tap into the support that family and friends can offer by sharing your accomplishments.

✦ **Visualize your goals.** Imagine yourself riding on that bike, fitting into your favorite jeans, nailing that new dance combo, or hitting that ball over the net. Positive visualization helps us to get over our fears or doubts.

✦ **Change your mind.** If negative thoughts sneak into your mind, replace them with positive ones. Envision the beautiful transformation taking place outside and inside, and be proud of yourself for making the effort to change your mind—and your life—for the better.

✦ **Celebrate small accomplishments.** If your goal was to walk a half mile, reward yourself when it's over by getting a massage or pedicure! Positive reinforcement gives us something to look forward to in the short term.

Moving Beyond Pain

Moving can be painful if you suffer from arthritis, fibromyalgia, low back pain, or other conditions. But in the long run it is therapeutic. Moving arthritic joints, for example, helps lubricate the joint surface, improves range of motion, and strengthens the muscles around the joint, which ultimately reduces pain. This is why bicycling is often recommended for those with knee arthritis. Similarly, stretching back muscles that have become stiff promotes healing.

Aqua therapy, aqua-aerobic classes, and swimming can offer a low-impact, pain-free way to strengthen your body. The warm water used in therapy pools relaxes tight muscles, and the buoyancy of the water decreases joint pressure. I've had many patients who were unable to walk due to debilitating back or knee pain participate in forty-five-minute aqua-aerobic classes without a trace of discomfort. If pain is limiting your ability to live dynamically, be sure to talk with your doctor or physical therapist and explore your exercise options. No matter what your disability or limitations, I am confident that a creative clinician can allow you to reap the miraculous benefits of exercise.

THE AGES AND STAGES OF FITNESS

Some people believe the frequency and intensity with which you exercise depends on your age and fitness level. You might be surprised to learn that perseverance is more important than either of these because our bodies have a remarkable ability to adapt and change.

Like our brain, our body is constantly changing. We have the ability to grow stronger with every step we take, and it's never too late to start taking control over our body. A woman named Ruth Rothfarb ran the Boston Marathon at age eighty-six and didn't even start running until age sixty-nine! She was eighty when she entered in her first marathon. British equestrian Lorna Johnstone was seventy years old when she competed at the 1972 Olympics. And at the ripe age of one hundred, Ruth Frith competed in the shot put at the World Master Games in Australia, which are open to athletes of all ages and abilities. Clearly these women are not limited by age, and they are role models for all of us. Remember, age is a state of mind, and we can change our bodies simply by changing the way we think. These women and other female athletes prove that the only limits we have are the ones that we place on ourselves.

Exercise Promotes Faster Healing

Researchers at the University of Illinois had mice run for thirty minutes for three days before and five days after receiving a skin wound. Healing times were compared with those that were not allowed to exercise. The study revealed mice that exercised healed faster than those that weren't allowed to run. It is thought that the increased blood flow from exercise speeds up healing time by delivering oxygen, nutrients, and specialized healing cells to the injured area. Yet another reason to move it!

BE THANKFUL

One of the gifts of practicing medicine has been the inspiration I get from my patients. Seeing life-threatening events and illnesses helps me to focus on what's truly important. Paralysis and loss of motor function are common ailments in neurologic conditions. For those who recover, there is a new wonder in simply raising an arm or taking a step. For those who do not, acceptance and coping are the hallmarks of healing. Seeing the determination of an amputee negotiating ski slopes, and the triumphant spirit of wheelchair participants in the Boston Marathon, is deeply moving and inspiring. For me their message rings loud and clear: If you possess the ability to move, in whatever way you can, revel in it! Don't wait for a catastrophic illness to appreciate and indulge in the joy of movement.

While it is a true accomplishment to compete in a marathon, Newbies needn't be satisfied with simply cheering from the sidelines. Your goal might be a bit less lofty, but the idea of crossing your own personal finish line should be a means for celebration! The simple act of putting one foot in front of another is nothing less than a miracle, because it is a prime example of how our mind and body work in perfect, intelligent unison.

Walking Keeps Your Brain Young

Science has proven again and again that walking is good for your brain. One recent six-month study compared a group of seniors who walked for one hour, three times a week, with seniors who took a one-hour stretch-and-tone class three times a week. Brain MRIs were done on both groups at the beginning and at the end of the study. Significant increases in brain volume were seen in the walkers but not in the stretch-and-tone group.

In another study, published in the *Archives of Internal Medicine*, researchers also concluded that the more you walk, the better it is for your brain. They tested the cognitive abilities of 5,925 women sixty-five and older. The women were tested once and then again six to eight years later. Those who walked the least, about one block per day, were more likely to develop cognitive decline compared to those who walked an average of twenty-five blocks a day.

Consider the landmark achievement of learning how to walk. Infants begin to hone their motor skills as soon as they emerge from the womb. Initially their movements are jerky and appear erratic. When they squirm, wriggle, and feel their bodies move for hours on end, an incredible amount of learning takes place in the brain. Sensory receptors throughout the body, including those in the muscles and joints, are stimulated and relay information back to the brain. Motor pathways are forged and refined over time, allowing us eventually to stand and take a step. Of course, walking eventually leads to running, which kids do with a playful sense of abandon.

As adults we need to recapture that childlike joy of movement. You don't have to be in a playground to get your adrenaline flowing and to experience the excitement that comes with having fun being active!

Have a Booty Shake

n addition to all the beautiful brain benefits you get from aerobic exercise, physical exertion has been shown to suppress appetite longer than nonaerobic activity. So have a booty shake instead of a milk shake and watch the calories and the pounds disappear.

BOOST YOUR INTENSITY

Whatever form of activity you choose, picking up the pace and increasing your heart rate will boost your brain power and improve your health and stamina. Maximal heart rates, the fastest speed your heart can safely pump during exercise, and target heart rates, the rate in which your heart and lungs get the most benefit, vary tremendously based on age, fitness, and individual physiology. Like the brain, our heart changes in size and efficiency based on how it is used. By exercising both your heart and brain over time, your maximal and target heart rates can change. As long as you've gotten your doctor's okay to exercise, the following simple guide is an easy way to gauge your intensity level while you exercise:

+ **Mild intensity.** There is minimal change in your breathing. You can easily carry on a conversation while you exercise.

✦ **Moderate intensity.** You are breathing faster and need to pause during conversation. You might have worked up a light sweat.

✦ **High intensity.** You are breathing faster, sweating profusely, and unable to carry on a conversation.

CALORIE-BURNING MYTH BUSTER

Perhaps even more confusing than calculating target heart rates is trying to figure out how many calories you are burning during physical activity. While there are many estimates about how many calories you burn while doing housework or even while kissing, the truth is the number of calories you burn with any activity depends upon your weight, your fitness level, and the intensity with which you are performing the activity. And don't believe those "calories burned" estimates on cardio machines—they are notoriously inaccurate.

I advise my patients to use the intensity scale above to estimate how much energy they are expending and to try to increase the time spent doing higher-end intensity activities every week. For example, if you are a Newbie walking fifteen minutes three times a week at a mild intensity, try interspersing intervals of moderate intensity the following week. Start out slowly with ten- to thirty-second intervals at a faster clip, and let your body recover before you try it again. Gradually increase the duration, intensity, and frequency of your physical activity. As your stamina increases, you can incorporate spurts of energetic intervals into your daily life. Try it the next time you're cleaning the house, walking the dog, or raking leaves.

Move to the Music

One way to increase your pulse is to listen to upbeat music while you move. A study conducted by Christopher Capuano, Ph.D., at Fairleigh Dickinson University, New Jersey, found that subjects who listened to music while exercising lost twice as much weight as those who did not. Dr. C. I. Karageorghis, a sports and exercise psychologist at Brunel University, UK, says there are several ways that music enhances performance in exercise and sports. It can divert attention away from fatigue or discomfort, it can increase our level of arousal, and when the rhythm of the song is in synch with our movement, we exert ourselves more strenuously. Whether you're striding around the block, gardening, making dinner, or vacuuming, plug in your iPod and groove as you move!

DYNAMIC LIVING FOR GONNABES

Gonnabes want to exercise, but they don't because they feel that they are too tired, too busy with work and child care duties, or too depressed, or too busy to find the time. They tend to exercise in fits and starts, running each day for a week or so, until some stressful event in their life gives them the excuse to "temporarily" put their exercise on hold. The fact is, if you are too tired or too stressed out to get up and get moving, these are the precise reasons why you need to start "playing-out." Regular exercise will ultimately give you more energy, help relieve your stress, and improve your mood. These benefits are free, immediate, and they don't require a prescription or even visits to a therapist. Duke University researchers found that performing moderate-intensity cardio three times a week was as effective as the antidepressant Zoloft at relieving depression.

According to the latest U.S. government guidelines on exercise, adults should do two hours and thirty minutes a week of moderate-intensity exercise, or one hour and fifteen minutes (seventy-five minutes) a week of vigorous aerobic activity, or the equivalent combination of both. It is best to spread this out over the course of the week, and if necessary, you can even break it up into ten-minute intervals. You can get even more health benefits from five hours (three hundred minutes) a week of moderate activity, or two hours and thirty minutes of high-intensity activity. Additionally, adults should do muscle-strengthening exercise for two or more days a week. Think about how much time you spend doing things that you can cut out, such as watching TV or texting. I'm not suggesting you give up TV and throw away your smart phone, just substitute one thirty-minute reality show with thirty minutes of exercise.

Making time for physical activities is just as important as brushing your teeth, eating, and showering—and, like your personal hygiene habits, it will improve your health, make you look better, give you more energy, and potentially add years to your life.

TIMING IS EVERYTHING

I understand that it's difficult to get yourself moving when you're working, hungry, or tired, or the kids need to be ferried to their music lessons. This is why timing is everything when it comes to scheduling your Dynamic Living program. Some people are larks, and some are owls, and you probably know which one you are. If you're a lark, rise with the sun, especially before the rest of the family stirs, and do your playouts in the morning. Night owls might prefer exercising after work or after everyone is safely tucked into bed.

Research suggests that it takes new exercisers about three to five weeks to make their sessions a habit. And hitting the road at dawn or dusk doesn't mean you'll miss out on sleep either. Studies show that cardio activity can actually make you sleep better. Let your biological clock and lifestyle dictate your Dynamic Living routine.

Be creative about inserting bursts of activity into your daily round as a way to boost your fitness even if your schedule is chock-full of obligations. Throughout my medical training there were thirty-six-hour shifts when I couldn't leave the hospital. Of course, because of the physical, intellectual, and emotional demands of my work, I needed the benefits of exercise more than ever. So I decided to make the hospital my gym. During my nights on call, I would strap on ankle weights under my scrubs and take the multiple flights of stairs up and down to the emergency room. I did sit-ups in the on-call room and interspersed brisk walks throughout the day. Although I now have much more control over my schedule, there are still times when it's jam-packed. On these days, I find it helpful to use the suggestions below.

Multitask

We all know that women are great at multitasking, so why not apply your gender-given talent to your Dynamic Living routine. Need time to come up with a new promotion plan for work? Do it while you're walking, running, cycling, or on the treadmill. Need to problem solve an issue one of your kids is having at school? Some of our best ideas and solutions come when we are in the midst of doing other things, so whether it's vacuuming or running with your Baby Jogger, use your playout time productively.

Be Your Own StairMaster

No time to go to a gym? Take the stairs instead of the elevator. To sweat even more, take them two at a clip. Running up and down the stairs for ten minutes four times a day makes an excellent daily cardio playout.

Run Errands

On days when you are going to be running errands and on the move, dress appropriately for your playout. Wear a good pair of running shoes and zip through the mall, grocery store, or farmer's market. Strap on some ankle weights to increase the benefits. (Most can be hidden under yoga pants, but if you're wearing shorts, tell anyone who asks that "it's the latest fitness fashion!")

Be an Active Soccer Mom

Don't sit on the sidelines while your kids are playing soccer or softball. Whatever your child's sport of choice, taking a few spins around the field or court while you watch your kids play is better for your brain and body than cheering from the bleachers.

Stay on Your Toes

Instead of eating at your desk, take a walk around the block and enjoy lunch at a local park, gallery, or mall. Enlist a colleague or your Beautiful Brain Buddy to go with you. Stand up and walk around as much as possible when talking on the phone or dictating. Instead of sending an e-mail to a colleague, deliver your message in person.

Jump for Joy

Jumping rope is one of the easiest and cheapest ways to get in a good cardio playout anytime and anywhere. You can bring a jump rope with you when traveling for business or pleasure, and you can even do it while you're watching TV. Make sure you buy a good pair of athletic shoes, however, because jumping rope can put a lot of stress on your calf and other leg muscles. You'll be sore the first few times you do it, but your heart and brain will be jumping for joy!

Choose an Activity That Stirs Your Passion

Even if you don't have the time to indulge in regular exercise, it's important to have at least one athletic pursuit that you love to keep you motivated to move. If horseback riding is your passion, plan a dude ranch vacation and saddle up. If you like to dance, go for a night of clubbing, two-stepping, or however you like to kick it. If golf excites you, book a tee time when the kids are away at camp. This way, you will stay connected to what you enjoy doing most and keep up your determination (and skills), which will help you stay in shape. And when the time comes for you to indulge more often—you'll be ready!

DYNAMIC LIVING FOR TRAINIACS

I realize that I don't have to tell you to get out there and move, because fitness is your drug of choice. (Thanks again, endorphins!) For Trainiacs, it's okay to indulge in "workouts," because you probably love your work, including the kind you do on your feet. You are type A, for athlete, and what you want to know is how to exercise harder and more efficiently, without the risk of injury. So here are some ways for you to safely step up your workouts.

Cross Train Your Brain

Many women perform the same exercise routine week in and week out and complain that they are not getting any results. As Albert Einstein once said, "Doing the same thing over and over again and expecting a different result is the definition of insanity." Not only does this get boring, but it's not developing your body and brain as a whole. Our muscles quickly adapt to a routine workout and are no longer challenged. Once again, the brain is constantly changing as we learn and do new things, so engaging in a different physical activity will also strengthen new neural circuits.

The muscles we use when running are different from those we use in racquetball. Judging the angle and speed of a moving target is a complex visual function that challenges multiple brain areas. Likewise the balance skills used to ride a bicycle are different from those we use in advanced yoga. Activities that require precise rhythm and timing, such as rowing, diving, or dancing, will develop your brain in different ways.

Trying diverse activities is not only good for your brain but will also help you get better at your favorite sport. If you're a tennis player, play singles instead of doubles, or play with a more expert partner who will fire up your neurons as well as your game. If you enjoy skiing every season, try doing it on water instead of on the mountains. Snap into a snowboard and see how that feels. Go swimming as well as spinning. Knowing how to blade makes it easier to learn how to ice-skate (and vice versa), and doing yoga will help you when you cycle or do other sports.

Interval Training

Whatever sport or activity you choose, there is a natural up-and-down cadence in exertion that varies in intensity. When kayaking, for example, a steady current may give way to a strong eddy. In tennis, the calm before a serve is followed by a burst of energy. Revving up the intensity of our workouts increases the cardiovascular benefits of movement. If you run, try taking a different route, go outside instead of in the gym, or challenge yourself with variable terrain. Running against the wind will make you push harder, and taking a steeper hill or path that is uneven will challenge your balance. When running on a treadmill, increase your speed or incline level to simulate going uphill and then take a breather.

Varying the intensity of your workouts will get you the most health and brain bang for your buck. Take it up a notch for whatever period of time you feel comfortable, then slow it down until your heart rate and breathing recover. Do this intermittently during the activity and again whenever it feels right for you. How long and how hard you rev it up to, and the time it takes for your heart rate and breathing to recover, depend on your physical condition. But over time this is guaranteed to improve your fitness level.

Meet to Compete

If you are a Trainiac with a competitive spirit, signing up for a triathlon (a swim, bike, and running race) will get your juices flowing. Last summer I watched my husband and son compete in a local competition, and I was impressed by how many women were participating. Having grown up in a time when there were few options for female athletes, I was truly moved. I began training the next day. Two months later, I completed my first bona fide race, and although my time was not remarkable, the experience was awesome. Many sports clubs now offer training programs for biathlons and triathlons, or you can form your own training group. Athletic contests are springing up all across the country, and some are for women only! If these kinds of races are not for you, but you enjoy competition, consider sports like softball, tennis, soccer, racquetball, or paddleball. The possibilities are limitless. The winner can take the others out for a postgame celebration.

Thrill Sports

Trainiacs thrive on the adrenaline rush, and nothing is more powerful than the need for speed. To that end, put on the proper gear and head toward the mountains for some downhill thrills (and possibly spills), strap on some skates and go blading around the park (watch out for the cars if you head onto the streets), or wax up your board and go surfing. The name of the game is fun, and if you love it you will probably make it a regular part of your fitness regimen. Whatever you do, be absolutely sure to protect your head with the proper safety gear, including a helmet. Unlike bones and joints, which can be mended, brain and spinal cord injuries are often permanent. You have only one brain, and it must last you a lifetime!

Heads Up!

As I mentioned in the previous step, your brain has the consistency of Brie cheese, and it floats within cerebrospinal fluid that cushions it from the bumps and dings of everyday life. Although protected by the skull, it is nevertheless vulnerable to injury, which can cause bleeding, bruising, and damage to delicate brain tissue, the degree of which depends on the severity of the force. Concussions occur far more often than most people realize, and you don't have to lose consciousness to sustain a brain injury. Any blow to the head or violent head movement that causes a change in brain function, whether you have been knocked out or just feel "dazed," is a concussion.

Common symptoms include confusion, dizziness, loss of balance, the inability to think clearly, memory problems, headache, nausea, change in behavior, ringing in the ears, and loss of consciousness. It's important to understand that even a mild concussion means that the brain has been injured. If there is loss of consciousness or if symptoms persist or worsen, call an ambulance. When in doubt, call your doctor.

If you have suffered a concussion, no matter how mild, you must try to avoid a second injury while the brain is healing. Second Impact Syndrome, as it is called, has been the cause of death in young athletes who have sustained multiple concussions. There is also a growing body of evidence that people who have had multiple concussions have an increased risk of developing dementia, including Alzheimer's.

Women have more concussions than men, according to studies of high school and college athletes. While researchers don't know why this is, they suspect that it is because women have smaller heads and weaker necks than men, which increases the forces acting on the brain. Again, please protect your brain by wearing helmets and by using the proper equipment for biking, skating, skiing, snowboarding, and other fast-moving sports. Make sure you are fully outfitted for whatever activity you are doing and that you understand the manufacturer's instructions and guidelines. And while you're driving to wherever you are going to work out, wear a seat belt!

Walk the Walk

Did you know that the way you walk reveals a great deal about your health? When I invite patients into my office, I watch as they rise from the waiting room chair and walk toward me. Stooping forward or to one side implies muscle weakness and poor flexibility. I also pay special attention to stride—how easily each leg clears the floor, the length of each step, and whether their steps are symmetric. Pain in a joint or muscle will result in the patient favoring a limb, which creates a tense, uneven motion as they walk.

Similarly, if someone suffers from balance problems, they are apt to take short, cautious strides, which leads to decreased flexibility, strength, and endurance over time. Walking that is effortful and causes heavy breathing suggests poor cardiovascular fitness. By the time my patients reach the threshold of my office, I often have a good sense of what their diagnosis will be.

Whatever the underlying cause, I regularly recommend working with a physical therapist. When you walk with grace and confidence you exude a newfound sense of well-being and energy. With proper balance training, stretching, and strengthening, you will be taking the first few steps toward Dynamic Living in your stride!

BE WELL ROUNDED

Consider how running, yoga, and weight lifting complement one another. Running improves aerobic capacity, which in turn will enhance your endurance when weight lifting or through a long yoga class. The increased flexibility from yoga will lengthen your running stride, allowing you to run smoother and faster. Your improved flexibility will also increase your range of motion while weight lifting, which in turn will make your muscles stronger. Lifting weights increases muscle strength, which will make you a stronger runner and improve your endurance and balance when maintaining strenuous yoga postures. All of these activities reinforce one another, and the total benefit is much greater than the sum of its parts. Aerobic capacity is only one part of the fitness equation. To truly reap the benefits of a healthy body, weight training and flexibility are also essential.

USE IT OR LOSE IT!

About ten years ago when I was on a ski vacation, I tore my ACL (anterior cruciate ligament)—one of the four major ligaments in the knee. I was placed in a knee immobilizer that extended from my upper thigh to my midcalf. When it was removed three days later, I was shocked to find that my quadriceps (the front thigh muscle) had virtually disappeared! As a physician, I should have been aware of how quickly atrophy ensues when a muscle is not used, but I was surprised by how dramatic the change was in only a few short days.

The medical term for this withering away of a muscle is called "disuse atrophy." It is profound when there is complete immobilization of a muscle. (If you've ever been in a cast, you know how thin your arm or leg can become when it comes off.) Unfortunately, muscle atrophy can also occur when we decrease our level of activity and with age. In fact, the generalized weakness we experience after being laid up in bed with the flu is due to muscle deconditioning. This effect can be seen in children as well as adults, but the older we are the longer the recovery can take.

Muscles are designed to move, and they need to in order to stay strong. And just like our brain, our muscles are constantly changing. They are molded by the stimulation they receive from the nerves that control their activity. How often and how strenuously they are used determines their contour and tone. As we get older, we tend to lose muscle over time. Although building muscles takes much longer than it takes for a muscle to break down, the good news is that muscles of any age—even when we're ninety—become stronger with use, and weight training is the single most effective way to keep your muscles strong. Empowering your muscles will:

◆ Protect your joints from injury.

◆ Improve your balance.

◆ Relieve neck, back, and other joint pain.

◆ Allow you to move better whatever the activity.

◆ Burn more calories. Gaining muscle mass increases our metabolic rate. Even at rest muscles burn many more calories than fat!

◆ Make your bones stronger and prevent osteoporosis.

◆ Give you a psychological boost, because a strong woman is a confident woman!

WOMEN HOLD UP HALF THE SKY

It has been said that women hold up half the sky, a poetic nod to our contributions to the world, but we have also been called "the weaker sex." While there is no biological doubt that men are physically stronger, this doesn't mean that women can't do their part and pull their weight. And the best way to improve one's muscle strength is through resistance training or weight lifting. Fortunately, strength training can be short and sweet, and results can be achieved by doing it just twice a week.

Having the proper form is essential for avoiding injury, so it is worth your while to work with a physical therapist, trainer, or experienced lifter, at least in the beginning. If you don't belong to a gym, get a DVD that will instruct you on form and working the different muscle groups. Whether you lift at home or in a gym, it's a good idea to have a professional review your form periodically. It's easy to fall into bad habits, and lifting weights incorrectly can do more harm than good and possibly result in injury.

It is also important to develop opposing muscle groups in a balanced way. Otherwise you can throw your whole body out of whack. For example, many women have weak upper back muscles (those between the shoulder blades), causing them to stoop forward with poor posture. This problem becomes compounded if you focus on building up your pectoralis (chest) muscles and neglect your upper back. Once again, having a professional review your workout is worth the investment.

Resistance training or weight lifting should not be done on consecutive days. After working your muscles with weights, small muscle tears occur, which need time to heal. This is the natural process of how muscle growth takes place and what gives us that mild soreness the day after doing weight lifting. You should feel a "good soreness" that is mild and resolves in a day or two. If you are feeling severe pain during or after weight lifting, stop immediately, because you are putting yourself at risk of injury. Weight lifting should challenge your muscles, but it should never be painful.

Free weights (the kind you can hold in your hands) work multiple muscle groups at once. For this reason, they are more efficient and it will take you much less time to achieve your goals than using the machines in a gym. For each major muscle group, eight to twelve repetitions are recommended. In just fifteen minutes, you can perform an adequate resistance workout that will keep your muscles strong. To get the most out of your workout, use a variety of strength exercises to target different muscle groups, and vary the size of the weights and the number of repetitions. Not only does it make your training more interesting, but it also keeps your muscles guessing. If you don't want to use equipment, you can also use your body's own resistance by doing push-ups, sit-ups, squats, and lunges with or without weights as another great way to increase your strength. You might also consider mountain, rock, or wall climbing; advanced yoga; and Pilates, all of which will improve your strength (and flexibility).

The Intelligence of Movement

Have you ever started to lift what you think is a heavy suitcase only to find that it is empty and unexpectedly light? Without consciously thinking about it, your brain has estimated the expected weight of the suitcase, which dictated how many motor units in your arm muscles needed to contract, and the force needed to lift the case. Similarly muscles in your back, abdomen, and legs were instructed to contract in preparation for the heavy load and to keep you upright and counterbalanced. This sophisticated planning of a simple motor activity is an example of how precise, calibrated, and complex our motor system is.

BE FLEXIBLE

As with the muscles that atrophy with disuse, if we do not move our muscles through their full range of motion, they will eventually become shorter and tighter. When we experience pain, whether it is in our neck, back, arm, or leg, it is natural to restrict our movements. But if the underlying problem is not corrected, it will lead to decreased flexibility in that body part.

Another common cause of stiffness comes from not stretching. While cardio exercise is essential for maintaining our brain function, flexibility is equally important for maintaining our body's ability to move with youthful fluidity. Stretching should never be painful when done correctly; in fact, it should feel good. Savor the feeling of lengthening your muscles when stretching and strive to increase your flexibility gradually. Never do more than your body can handle. Ideally, you should do some type of stretching every day. Just a few minutes will do the trick. Here are some fun ways to fit stretching into your daily physical regimen.

Stretching for Newbies

There are a variety of classes that focus on stretching and flexibility, including Pilates and yoga. Start with beginner level classes and always talk to the instructor beforehand to let her know you're new. You can also practice stretching on your own at home with a DVD that shows you how to use proper form and alignment.

Stretching for Gonnabes

There are many ways to work stretches into your daily life. When drying your hair, flip your hair over and touch your toes. Try putting your leg onto a sturdy desk or countertop. Keep it as straight as possible and don't do more than you can handle comfortably. (Be sure the floor and counter are dry to avoid slipping.) If you can't straighten your leg without bending your knee, go to a lower height.

Counter stretching is also a great way to lengthen your back muscles. Simply stand in front of a sink that is well rooted into the floor. Grasp the front edge of the sink in the same way you would hold on to a ballet barre and round your back up like a cat stretching, then bend forward until your spine is flat. Or, while sitting at the office or at home, round forward in your chair and hang your head between your knees to stretch out your spine. Reach for the sky and stretch your arms and torso; bend to the side, arch your back. This should all feel good, so if you experience any pain, stop immediately. Watch an instructional DVD on yoga or Pilates, or take a class. Both will improve your flexibility, which is a great complement to any aerobic activity.

Stretching for Trainiacs

In addition to adding more stretching to your fitness routine, I suggest you hire a professional trainer who will challenge your flexibility and push you to a new level. You will find that daily stretching will improve your overall athletic performance. Upper level yoga, Pilates studios that have machines, and dance classes are a few ways to go.

GET READY TO MAKE OVER YOUR MIND

Now that you've worked (or played) to transform your body, it's time to relax, let go, and make over your mind. We will address how stress wreaks havoc on your brain and appearance, and show you how to use the Relaxation Response (a proven stress-reducing technique) and other empowering skills to control your thoughts. Making over your mind not only protects you from memory loss by making your brain healthier, but it also helps you to look and feel better so you can fully enjoy the gorgeous gift of life. So get ready to make over your mind and get one step closer to that beautiful brain and beautiful you!

Make Over Your Mind

Think left and think right and think low and think high.
Oh, the thinks you can think up if only you try!

—DR. SEUSS

From the moment we open our eyes in the morning to the time we fall asleep at night, a constant stream of thoughts flows through our mind. It's been estimated that we have twelve thousand thoughts per day, although some say the number is closer to sixty thousand. One way to figure this out for yourself is to actually count the number of thoughts you have over a thirty-second period and then do the math. Of course, just the thought of counting your thoughts would affect the results. If you have children, you can probably add an extra hundred thoughts per child! The bottom line is—no one really knows how many thoughts we have per day, but we can all agree that it's a remarkable number.

On days when we are busy, our stream of consciousness is more like a deluge: "I forgot to pick up milk last night . . . I should stop for some coffee on my way to work . . . Today's Mom's birthday, I better give her a call . . . The car's been making a funny noise, wonder what's wrong with it? . . . Why does everything break down just when I don't have the time? . . . I need to do the laundry soon . . . What am

I going to make for dinner?" Now compare these types of thoughts to those we might have on the third or fourth day of a tropical vacation. "Gee, these sheets are so silky . . . Look how blue the ocean is . . . I love the scent of ocean air . . . It feels like seventy-five degrees already . . . What a gorgeous day!"

Although we can't spend our life on vacation (as wonderful as that might sound), we *can* control the floodgates of our mind. No matter how many thoughts we have each day, we can learn to stem the flow from a raging torrent to a gentle stream. And we can learn to control the quality of those thoughts, replacing nonproductive and destructive ones with those that are empowering and life enhancing. This step is about "making over" your mind by taking control of your thoughts. By doing this, you can literally restructure your brain, which will profoundly improve your mental clarity, moods, and every aspect of your life, including the way you present yourself to the world.

It starts by being aware of what your mind is up to and tapping into the power of neuroplasticity—your brain's ability to make new connections. By refusing to think negative, self-defeating thoughts, the pathways that processed those thoughts will weaken and fade away like a trail in the woods that has become overgrown with weeds through disuse. Instead I want your thoughts to travel along new pathways that will serve you better. In some cases, we might need to forge new, healthier mental pathways. In others, we might just need to clear out the brush that has accumulated.

In the same way that your physical strength and flexibility improve with regular exercise, thinking optimistic thoughts on a regular basis strengthens and reinforces healthy mental pathways. Making over your mind will alleviate stress, improve your mood, and protect you from memory loss, which allows your intellect and creativity to blossom and transforms your appearance. Instead of looking frazzled, overwhelmed, and depressed, you will experience an inner calm and joy that others will notice.

In this step, you will learn how to change the way you think using the scientifically proven methods of the Relaxation Response, pioneered by the internationally renowned Harvard cardiologist Dr. Herbert Benson, and by learning the basics of cognitive behavioral therapy (CBT). As Buddha once said, "We are what we think." By learning how to relieve stress and rethink and respond differently to the negative experiences in your daily life, you can tap into the true power of your mind!

You will also learn how to emerge from a state of "mindlessness"— that fog we sometimes find ourselves in when we are not truly present or our mind is wandering. It can help when we are suffering from so-called Mommy Brain or Senior Moments; when we don't remember the names of the people we are introduced to; when we forget the reason we walked into a room; or when we can't retrieve a bit of information that is frozen on the tip of our tongue.

Mindfulness, which has its roots in Eastern philosophy, is being aware of what we are thinking. This not only makes us sharper but also ultimately determines how we feel. We alone are responsible for the thoughts that we think, and it is within our power to change the way we think. No one else can do this for us.

STRESSED (INSIDE) OUT

Before we work on changing our negative thoughts, you should be aware of the toll stress takes on our health and our appearance. Although stress is an unavoidable fact of life, when we are continually "stressed-out" it ages our cells, which is why stress makes us look older than our years.

As we talked about in the last step, aging takes place within the individual cells that make up our body. Remember the "telomeres" that look like the tips of shoelaces and prevent the chromosomes inside our cells from becoming unraveled or frayed? The shorter our telomeres, the faster our cells are aging.

Research by Nobel Prize winner Dr. Elizabeth Blackburn showed how stress accelerates cellular aging. Dr. Blackburn compared the telomere length of two groups of mothers: One group had healthy children, while the other group had chronically ill children. As she suspected, the mothers who cared for a chronically ill child had shorter telomeres. In other words, the stress of caring for a sick child was making the mothers' cells age faster.

Why are our cells so important in determining how we look? If our cells are not aging well on the inside, it will show on the outside. Our skin will wrinkle, the connective tissue that supports our skin will sag, and our hair will become thin and lackluster. Our emotional well-being and our ability to handle stress are therefore intimately linked to our appearance.

This reciprocal relationship between mind-set and skin disorders has even created a new subspecialty called psychodermatology. For example, stress can manifest itself in one's appearance by making the skin more sensitive. It can trigger breakouts of psoriasis (a patchy, itchy rash), rosacea (redness), acne, seborrhea, herpes, and other skin conditions. Stress can also cause hair loss, brittle nails, and excessive perspiration. Learning to manage stress and improve your sense of well-being by making over your mind will make you more beautiful, both inside and out!

Brain Stress

It is no surprise that chronic stress ages us, but we now understand that stress also physically damages the brain. Cortisol, the so-called stress hormone, has been shown in animal studies to actually kill off neurons in the hippocampus, the brain's memory center. Animals under chronic stress have smaller hippocampi, and there is reason to believe the same holds true for humans. A study from the Rush Alzheimer's Disease Center in Chicago showed that people prone to distress were 2.4 times more likely to develop Alzheimer's than persons who were not. Many other studies support the notion that those who suffer from anxiety and depression also have an increased risk of Alzheimer's and stroke.

THE STRESS RESPONSE

When we perceive a threat to our physical or psychological well-being, we activate the stress response. This triggers the release of the "fight or flight" hormones and cortisol, which allowed our ancestors to cope with the dangers of warring tribes or fearsome animals. When these hormones put our brain on high alert, our attention improves and we become acutely aware of the world around us. Our heart rate and blood pressure shoot up, blood flow to the heart and muscles increases, and blood sugar and lipid levels rise to boost our energy supply.

When we are fleeing from a burning building or fighting off an attacking dog, the stress response serves us well. It is our body's "natural alarm system," and it is designed to help us mentally and physically confront the situation at hand. But this overdrive system is meant to be short-lived, lasting only minutes to hours. When the stress is over, the alarm should shut off and our body should return to normal. Problems arise, however, when the stress response lasts for days, months, or longer. If we have a stressful lifestyle or if we regularly feel stressed, the level of cortisol in our blood will remain high. This takes a toll on our brain and body.

High cortisol levels are associated with hypertension, diabetes, high cholesterol, and abdominal obesity. Do these notorious Brain Beauty Burglars sound familiar? When we are under chronic stress, persistently high cortisol levels make us feel moody and impair our concentration and memory. Chronic stress can weaken the immune system, making us more prone to illness and blood clotting.

Stress can also affect our appetite, causing us to eat more so-called comfort foods that might lead to obesity. (If you've ever polished off a pint of Ben & Jerry's after a breakup or a particularly stressful day, you know what I'm talking about.) This is called "stress eating." For others, chronic stress causes nausea and unhealthful weight loss. And as we all know, stress disrupts our sleep, compounding our poor concentration and fatigue and setting in motion a vicious cycle. Fortunately there is a way to stop our body's alarm system and avoid the devastating effects of the stress response. Learning the Relaxation Response is an empowering tool that will allow you to turn off the stress response whenever the need arises.

THE RELAXATION RESPONSE

I've been fortunate to be at Harvard, where I work with some of the greatest minds in medicine. Dr. Herbert Benson is one of those great minds. Back in the seventies, he discovered a scientifically proven and effective way to relieve stress called the Relaxation Response (RR). His book of the same name has been a national best seller for decades. The RR doesn't require meditation classes or for you to be sequestered in a quiet room or isolation tank. It can be done at work, at home, while running, while doing tai chi or yoga, or while meditating or praying—it can be done anytime during your busy day. Starting out, it is best to find a quiet, comfortable setting to help you focus. With training, however, you can learn to calm your mind regardless of what is taking place around you.

According to Dr. Benson, you need only remember these two steps in order to elicit the Relaxation Response:

1. Select a word, sound, prayer, or thought that you find soothing or joyous. Repeat that word, sound, prayer, or thought and focus your mind in the moment.

2. When other, everyday thoughts intrude, let them go and concentrate once again on step one, which is repeating a word, sound, prayer, or thought.

Our brains are constantly running, so one of the hardest parts of the RR will be learning how to control your thoughts and focus your mind on a single word, thought, or sound. Clearing your mind is like emptying the recycle bin of old files on your computer or taking the clutter out of an overstuffed drawer. It's a cleansing process that makes us feel better in the end. When I first started the RR, I was unable to rein in my thoughts, but like any new skill, it took practice. Now I try to do it every day, and I'm happy to report that my ability to stay focused has dramatically improved.

Doing the relaxation technique will help to reverse or prevent stress. While we all know that our heart rate and blood pressure slow down when we relax, what you might not realize is how the RR can physically change your body and your brain. Dr. Benson's research in mind-body medicine showed how people could actually alter their white blood cells in just eight weeks by doing the RR for twenty minutes a day. (White blood cells are the ones that fight infections and cancers and mediate our body's natural response to injury.) In other words, by simply focusing our mind, we can reprogram our cells! While scientists are still not sure exactly how this works, it is clear that making the RR part of your way of life will benefit your brain, health, moods, and ultimately your appearance. And because stress accelerates aging, doing the RR regularly will help you naturally look and feel younger.

Practicing the Relaxation Response

First, find a place that is quiet, where you will have no distractions. You don't need to sit in a cross-legged lotus position with your back aching. Comfort is important—so find a position that works for you. Lying on the floor or sitting in a chair is just fine. Make sure that your body is aligned (this will keep you alert). The idea is to be relaxed but conscious. Choose a word, sound, or thought to repeat. Don't overthink this (remember, we are trying to clear our head, not clog it up), so just pick one and try it out. You can always change it the next time you do the RR.

When you're first starting out, go easy on yourself and try not to get frustrated if you don't get it right away. Whenever you have a random thought, just let it pass through your mind. Some people like to imagine their thoughts drifting down a river; some picture them as bubbles floating away. Try various techniques and find one that works for you. Let's give it a try. Close your eyes and:

+ Repeat your chosen word, sound, prayer, or thought.

+ When other thoughts intrude, let them drift away, as we discussed above, and continue to repeat your chosen word, sound, prayer, or thought.

+ After five minutes, open your eyes.

As I said, the more you practice this, the easier it will become and the longer you will be able to maintain this restful state of mind. It can be helpful to focus on your breathing—that is, concentrating on nothing but the sound of your breath as you inhale and exhale. You can also try picturing yourself in a peaceful setting. Discover what works best for you by trying different things. As with the interval training we talked about in the last step, your goal is to increase the duration and frequency of this mental exercise. As Dr. Benson's study showed, doing the RR for twenty uninterrupted minutes a day is a reasonable goal that has very promising results.

I found it helpful to start with just five minutes. And while this might sound strange, I would set the vibrate alarm on my cell phone. Otherwise I would be obsessing about how much time was passing, and it also allayed my concern that, once I got the hang of it, I would be lost in meditation for hours and be playing catch-up for the rest of the day! Over time, the ease with which I can slip into a place of relaxation within my own mind has significantly improved. Don't expect to master this in a few sessions. Be kind to your mind and give it the time it needs to develop this life-changing skill. Relaxation CDs can also be helpful, or you might want to try a meditation retreat or a class.

Once you become proficient, you can do the RR anywhere, even with your eyes open or while you are exercising (as long as repetitive movement is involved). You can do it while you're waiting in an impossibly long line at the bank or supermarket, while you're stuck in a traffic jam (eyes open, of course), during a turbulent flight, before an interview or presentation at work, before a new date, during an argument with your spouse—the possibilities are endless! Whatever it is that makes your heart pound, sweat pour, and pulse race, you can master the ability to calm your mind and acquire a powerful tool for creating peace and tranquility in your life.

SENSES AND SENSIBILITY

Everything we learn and every experience we have is relayed to our brain through our senses. Consider this: The only way new information gets into our brain is through what we see, hear, touch, taste, and smell. In fact our brain is programmed to monitor the constant stream of incoming sensory information. When this stream is cut off, as with prolonged sensory deprivation, our brain becomes confused, and we begin to hallucinate. This was discovered in studies using sensory deprivation tanks back in the fifties. More recently, research from University College, London, showed that when people are in a sensory deprivation room completely devoid of light and sound for as few as fifteen minutes, many experienced visual hallucinations, paranoia, and depression.

Similarly, partial obscuration of our senses can cause mental fogginess. The elderly who are visually impaired or are hard of hearing know this all too well. Medical students are sometimes asked to wear glasses smeared with Vaseline and sound-blocking headphones to help them empathize with these geriatric conditions. They also try walking around in thickly padded foam booties and gloves. Most report that they felt "out of it" and were unable to meaningfully engage with others. I know that I have trouble focusing mentally when I'm not wearing my contact lenses. It's not unusual for me to say, "Let me put my eyes in so I can hear you!"

Yet we often ignore the richness and beauty of the sensory information that surrounds us every day. As the saying goes, we must take the time to stop and smell the roses. Doing so will improve your mood as well as your mental clarity. When we are aware of the sensory information streaming into our brain, we are focused on the present. Because our brains can hold only one thought at a time, when we are in the moment we cannot possibly worry about the future or relive unpleasant memories of the past. Allowing your brain to experience the present more fully will strengthen your connection to the world and to those around you. In doing so, contentment and calm will resonate from within.

COME TO YOUR SENSES

When our senses are impaired it puts us out of touch with the world around us, while being in tune with our senses heightens our awareness and our mental clarity. Here are some suggestions for keeping yourself and your senses fine tuned.

Vision

One of the best ways to preserve your vision is to see an ophthalmologist (eye doctor) annually to check for vision problems. Many "hidden" eye diseases such as cataracts, macular degeneration, glaucoma, and diabetic retinopathy cause progressive visual loss over time. When caught early most of these conditions can be treated or controlled. Smoking and chronic conditions such as hypertension, diabetes, and vascular disease can increase the risk of eye diseases and visual loss.

Remember to wear sunglasses and hats, even in the winter when the glare from the snow can be bright, to protect your eyes from ultraviolet rays, which increase the risk of cataracts and macular degeneration. There are many fashionable shades on the market today, so adding this accessory can spice up your wardrobe. Plus, squinting causes wrinkles! And don't forget to wear safety goggles when doing yard work or other activities that might cause physical eye injury.

Hearing

The inner ear contains delicate "hair cells" that convert sound waves into electrical impulses that are transmitted by the auditory nerves into the brain. The brain interprets these impulses into sound. A very loud noise can destroy these specialized cells, causing instant deafness. Repeated exposure to loud noises over time can damage these hair cells, resulting in permanent hearing loss. From household appliances such as food processors, blenders, and garbage disposals, to MP3 players and traffic noise, sounds that exceed the eighty-decibel safety limit bombard us every day. If you have to raise your voice to be heard or if you can't hear someone two feet away, the noise level is too loud.

Carry earplugs with you at all times. Avoid sitting near speakers at concerts and in auditoriums, and turn down the volume when using headphones. Apple has software allowing iPod users to lock the volume at a specific decibel level. There are also volume-limiting headphones on the market, including LoudEnough, that can protect you and your children, whose young ears are especially vulnerable to noise trauma. Hearing damage can occur from both loudness and duration, so limit your exposure to loud music.

Touch

Our sense of touch originates in tiny nerve endings in the bottom layer of our skin called the dermis, which covers our body from head to toe. When stimulated, these nerve endings send impulses along peripheral nerves that are relayed up the spinal cord to the parts of the brain that interpret sensation. This allows us to feel the caress of a loved one's hand or the ground beneath our feet, and to discriminate between a nickel and a dime when we reach into our pocket.

Our sense of touch can be impaired by a condition called "neuropathy," which damages the nerves that relay sensory information to the brain. This commonly causes numbness and pain in the hands and feet. There are many causes of neuropathy, including diabetes, alcohol abuse, and vitamin deficiencies. It is reversible in some cases, and the discomfort can often be relieved by special medications. If you notice numbness or pain in your hands or feet, be sure to see your doctor.

Taste and Smell

These two senses are intimately linked, which is why our sense of taste is affected when our nose is congested. The fusion of taste and smell is also what gives food flavor. Imagine not being able to savor your food the next time you go out to a fine restaurant! Scientists say that 75 percent of what we call "taste" is actually due to smell. The most common causes of impaired taste and smell are allergies, colds, and irritants like cigarette smoke (yet another reason to stop smoking!).

SAVOR YOUR SENSES

One of the best ways to relax and allow your mind to be in the moment is to let your senses drink in the beauty around you. The following can be done along with the RR or on their own.

✦ **Smell the roses.** Place a beautiful flower in a vase and meditate on its singular beauty. Breathe in its fragrant, exquisite scent. Read Eckhart Tolle's book *The Power of Now*, in which he talks about intensifying one's awareness by taking "one conscious breath or looking, in a state of intense alertness, at a flower, so that there is no mental commentary running at the same time."

✦ **Candle meditation.** Light a single candle, preferably one of your favorite scents. Focus on the flickering flame.

✦ **Delight in a bath ritual.** Fill up the tub with warm water, add your favorite bubble bath, bath salts, or bath oils or create your own version with essential oils, herbs or flowers. Enjoy the warm, fragrant, silky soak, and then pat dry with soft, fluffy towels.

✦ **Breathe in the world.** Be attentive to the aromas and scents that permeate your surroundings. Can you identify the layers of scent that infuse your world? I realize this is harder to do if you live in a city where the smells are less than savory, which is why you need to take walks in the park or go to the countryside as much as possible.

The Cat Lover

After undergoing heart surgery, Mary began seeing cats walking around her hospital room. "I love cats and find them comforting," she told me, "but I also know this isn't normal." Upon further examination and questioning, she noted the cats always appeared on the right side of the room. They would linger for a few minutes and then vanish. My exam revealed that she had lost vision in her right visual field. When I asked her to focus on my nose and waved my fingers to her right she couldn't see them. She hadn't noticed this before.

A CAT scan (which stands for computerized axial tomography and has no relation to felines) of her brain revealed that she'd had a small stroke in the part of the brain that processes visual information. Most likely a small blood clot was released during her surgery and became lodged in an artery that supplies the visual cortex. The part of her injured brain that stores visual memories was triggering small seizures, which caused her to see cats. Within a day of starting seizure medication, the cats disappeared, and soon she was able to return home to her husband and her *real* furry friends.

THINK TALLER, YOUNGER, THINNER

People who are bored, tired, or uncomfortable often slouch, which is a physical reflection of what they are thinking and feeling. Those who stand erect, on the other hand, project confidence and optimism. When we slump, our belly protrudes and our body language conveys negative energy to those around us. We might as well wear a sign that says I DON'T FEEL GOOD ABOUT MYSELF. By simply standing up straight, you instantly express self-assurance and vibrancy. Nothing is more alluring and charismatic than a woman who radiates an aura of confidence and positive energy.

Remember how smiling, even if forced, can help nudge your brain toward feeling happy? The same goes for good posture, which will make you look and *feel* taller, thinner, younger, and more confident. It is also important to sit up straight when practicing the RR, because a straight spine keeps our mind alert and allows us to concentrate on positive, empowering thoughts.

I realize many of us spend countless hours slumped over a computer, lugging heavy purses, wearing backpacks, or ferrying children around on our hips—all of which contribute to bad posture and poor alignment. If you are not aware of your posture, look at those photos of you again to see the way you stand. Are your shoulders up to your ears? Is your lower back and stomach pushed forward? Does your chin jut out so you form the letter *C*? Aside from the back, neck, and muscle pain slouching causes, having good posture is energizing because it gives your lungs more room to expand. Proper alignment also improves your athletic performance and prevents injury and wear and tear on your joints over time.

As an experiment, curl your head and upper back forward (as if you were trying to touch your nose to your belly button) while standing or sitting in a chair. Try to take a deep breath. It's difficult to do, because your rib cage can't expand. Now stand or sit up and pretend there is a string attached to the top of your head, as if you were a marionette being pulled toward the ceiling. Take another deep breath. Feel the difference? This is oxygen traveling to your brain and throughout your body.

If we spend most of our day slumped forward, the muscles between the shoulder blades in the upper back will become weak and slack from not being used. Meanwhile, the muscles across the front of the chest and shoulders that are overworked will become shortened and tighter over time. If you are used to slouching, it will feel unnatural to stand up straight at first because your upper back muscles are weak and are not used to holding your back straight. At the same time, in order to straighten your upper back, the muscles in the front of your chest (pectoralis) must lengthen and stretch out. This might also feel uncomfortable at first. Fortunately the beauty of the human body is that it conforms to how we use it. Strengthening the muscles of your upper back and stretching the chest muscles will eventually make them stronger and longer, which will transform the way you look and how you present yourself to the world.

DR. MARIE'S ONE-MINUTE POSTURE PRESCRIPTION

Improving your posture begins with body awareness. Have your Beautiful Brain Buddy analyze your stance, and do the same for her. Remember the toddler song "Heads, Shoulders, Knees and Toes"? Just add the pelvis into the mix and that's everything you need to remember. The more frequently you realign your body throughout the day, the quicker good posture will become second nature. The following are my one-minute prescriptions for some of the most common posture problems. I suggest getting a DVD or using a trainer to learn proper form before doing some of these exercises.

Posture Problem: Protruding Head

Prescription: Slide your head back so it is balanced on top of your spine. Feel it lift up toward the sky, and focus on lengthening your neck. Use the marionette image that I described earlier. Stretch tight neck muscles by rolling your head gently from side to side, and strengthen upper back muscles by doing push-ups against the wall or on the floor with a level head and back, bottom down, and straight legs.

Posture Problem: Shoulders and Upper Back Are Slumped Forward

Prescription: Roll your shoulders back, lift your chest up, and squeeze your shoulder blades together and down toward your waist. Stretch tight chest muscles by clasping your hands behind your back while squeezing your shoulder blades together and pulling your hands down toward the floor. Strengthen upper back muscles by doing the exercises above.

Posture Problem: Protruding Abdomen and Arched Lower Back

Prescription: Tilt your pelvis up and pull your tailbone down. Imagine you are trying to zipper a tight pair of jeans. Do exercises that stretch tight low back muscles such as the "cat and cow" positions (get on hands and knees and alternatively round your back up toward the ceiling and lower your head; then reverse by arching your back and lowering your abdomen toward the floor). Loosen tight hamstrings by sitting upright on the floor with both legs out straight. Extend your arms toward your feet and bend at the waist as far as possible while keeping your knees straight. Do crunches to strengthen abdominal muscles. Lying on your back with your knees bent, clasp your hands behind your head and press your elbows back. Keeping your spine straight and elbows pressed back, slowly lift your head and shoulders off the floor, hold for three seconds, and then slowly roll back down.

Posture Problem: Your Knees and Ankles Turn In

Prescription: Adjust your weight over your feet and stand with your toes pointing straight ahead. Now rotate your knees and ankles so they too are pointing straight ahead. Do exercises that stretch inner thigh muscles, and strengthen outer thigh, ankle, and foot muscles (for example, side-to-side lunges and rising up and down on your toes with straight legs).

Deborah's Story

Deborah, a forty-five-year-old interior decorator, was suffering from daily headaches. The pain started in the back of her head and upper neck and radiated to her forehead. She had been working longer hours on a new project and figured it was due to stress. But when her headaches made it difficult for her to focus on her work, she became concerned that she might have a brain tumor, so she came to see me.

When I first met Deborah, I was struck by her worried expression. She told me that she had read about the symptoms of a brain tumor online and that this exactly matched her symptoms. I explained that headaches have many causes. As I examined Deborah, I noticed that her head jutted forward and her shoulders were slouched. I felt the back of her head and found she had marked tenderness at the base of her skull and the top of the neck. Everything else was normal.

I reassured Deborah that she did not have a brain tumor and that her headaches were actually triggered by her poor posture. You see, the average human head weighs about ten pounds, which is rather heavy compared to the rest of our body. We are designed to balance our heads on top of the spine—aligning it with our center of gravity. When our head juts forward, the muscles in our neck become strained trying to hold the weight of the head when it is off center, making it even heavier. The farther from center our head is held, the harder the neck muscles have to work. (Think about how much easier it is to hold a heavy bundle close to your body than in outstretched arms.) In Deborah's case, her neck muscles were so strained that it caused pain to radiate to her head.

After hearing this explanation, Deborah said, "You know, I feel better already." I wasn't surprised, because stress and worry can amplify pain. Although her headaches were caused by her bad posture, when she started worrying that she had a brain tumor, her pain became even more severe. I referred her to a physical therapist who taught her how to stretch and relax her tight neck muscles and gave her exercises to strengthen her upper back. She got an ergonomic workstation and learned how to maintain proper alignment while sitting. Deborah also started taking frequent breaks from work to get up, stretch, and move. Within a few weeks her headaches were gone.

Empowered Thoughts

One of the most sophisticated and exciting fields of neuroscience combines the power of the mind with technology. Quadriplegics (people who are paralyzed from the neck down) can now operate computers by using their thoughts. The computer learns to recognize an individual's thoughts as a specific pattern of brain activity, which is then relayed as a command. If thoughts can help those with special needs regain control of their bodies, just think of what the power of the mind can do for those of us who do not have these physical constraints.

MAKE OVER YOUR THOUGHTS

Now that you understand more about the power of your mind and how it can change the way you look and feel, it's time to examine the quality of your thoughts. As we've talked about earlier, the way we use our brain determines its structure. Every thought and experience produces changes. The brain you have at this moment is a product of the thoughts streaming through your mind and the experiences you've had throughout your life. And because we are creatures of habit, we get used to thinking and using our mind in the same way. The way we use our brain is the way we've *learned* to use our brain.

We don't question the negative thoughts and judgments that flow through our mind. And we often get stuck listening to a critical inner voice, which unconsciously determines the way we feel and behave. This not only affects our mood, but it also limits our ability to cope with stress. As author and motivational speaker Wayne Dyer said, "If you change the way you look at things, the things you look at change."

Using cognitive behavioral therapy (CBT) can help you overcome many of the problems that might be holding you back, including phobias, depression, poor self-esteem, mood swings, personality disorders, relationship difficulties, eating disorders, and anxiety. CBT is based on the idea that our *thoughts* cause our feelings and behaviors, rather than external things like people, situations, and events. It teaches us how to change the way we think so we can feel and act better, even if our situation does not change.

By using CBT we can learn how to listen to a new and improved inner voice. This kind of "thought makeover" is like turning to another radio station in your head. Instead of listening to the negative brain chatter that creates a harmful mind-set, you can tune in to a new station—one that transmits a healthier, calmer sense of self that has your best interests at heart. So how do we find this new station?

It begins by understanding that much of our stress has to do with how we perceive certain situations. Most of our negative thoughts contain distortions or exaggerations, which makes them invalid. We can rewire our brains and reduce our stress by replacing irrational thoughts with realistic, positive beliefs. The negative inner voice will eventually fade away as you continue to tune in to a calmer, more empowering voice that allows you to tap into your true potential.

CHANGE A NEGATIVE TO A POSITIVE

The following CBT steps can help you turn around your life by transforming your negative thoughts into positive ones. (I know you pessimists out there don't believe it, but it works!)

Step 1.
Recognize Negative Automatic Thoughts

When you feel anxious, depressed, or stressed, pause for a moment and identify your thoughts. Sometimes we have what are called "negative automatic thoughts" that seem to come out of nowhere and flash through our mind without us really being aware of them. They might seem plausible at the time, but they end up making you feel more anxious. Let's say you've invited a friend over for dinner and she hasn't returned your call. If you think "She must not like me anymore," you are having a negative automatic thought.

Step 2.
Challenge Negative Automatic Thoughts

A good way to challenge your negative thoughts is to understand that there are many different ways of looking at the same situation. Maybe your friend hasn't checked her voice or e-mail yet. Perhaps she's away on vacation. Or maybe she's so busy that she hasn't had time to respond. When you realize that your automatic thoughts contain thinking errors, you can stop jumping to upsetting conclusions.

Step 3.
Substitute Rational, Positive Thoughts and Beliefs

After you've learned how to identify your automatic negative thoughts and thinking errors, the next step is to substitute them with rational, positive thoughts and beliefs. A good substitute thought for the friend not responding to your invite might be: "I'm a good friend and I am kind to others, therefore others will be kind to me. If I don't hear from her by tomorrow, I'll call and make sure she is okay."

Common Negative Automatic Thoughts

Below are some other common types of negative automatic thoughts and examples of how you can change the way you think.

All-or-nothing thinking: Seeing things as black or white rather than as shades of gray. This thinking commonly uses words such as *always*, *never*, and *every*.

+ **Example:** You interview for a job but don't get it.

+ **Automatic negative thought:** "I'll never find a job."

+ **Substitute:** "Many other places are hiring. I have a great résumé and good contacts, so I'll find a job that's just right for me eventually."

Overgeneralizing: Assuming a negative event indicates a long-term pattern.

+ **Example:** You pick up your child late from day care.

+ **Automatic negative thought:** "I'm a bad mother."

✦ **Substitute:** "My child is well cared for and will not be traumatized by this. I love my child and I'm usually on time picking her up. I am a good mother."

Believing "should" statements: You live your life by a rigid set of rules, setting yourself up for disappointment and guilt.

✦ **Example:** You are a lawyer, and you believe that in order for something to be done right you must do it yourself. When you show up in court to defend an important case, your assistant brings the wrong file.

✦ **Automatic negative thought:** "I should have brought the file myself. If you want something done right, you have to do it yourself."

✦ **Substitute:** "Doing everything myself is unrealistic. This has happened to many lawyers before. I will simply request a brief postponement and send the assistant back for the correct file."

Dwelling on the negatives: Focusing on the negatives prevents you from enjoying the positive things that occur in life.

✦ **Example:** You're hosting a dinner party and you overcook the entrée.

✦ **Automatic negative thought:** "I've destroyed the meal— the evening is ruined!"

✦ **Substitute:** "The rest of the meal is so good, and my friends will understand. They are here for the company, not perfection. It will be a lovely evening."

Catastrophizing: Assuming that the worst is bound to happen in stressful situations.

+ **Example:** Your child hasn't come home on time; she's fifteen minutes late.

+ **Automatic negative thought:** "My daughter has been kidnapped or she was in a car accident!"

+ **Substitute:** "I trust my child. She makes good choices. This happened before and there was a perfectly reasonable explanation. I'm sure she'll call or show up soon. I'll give her a few more minutes and then call her cell phone."

Woe is me: You fail to take responsibility for your problems. When bad things happen, you usually feel like a victim.

+ **Example:** You never bothered to back up your computer files. Your computer crashes after you open a virus-ridden e-mail from a friend.

+ **Automatic negative thought:** "This wouldn't have happened if my friend hadn't sent that e-mail. Now I have to buy a new computer, and it's her fault."

+ **Substitute:** "I should have backed up my computer or installed virus protection. My friend didn't know she was sending me a virus. I'll make sure I'm protected in the future."

Dismissing the positives: You dismiss positive experiences and have trouble taking in compliments because you believe they don't count or they are untrue.

+ **Example:** You arrive at a party wearing your favorite dress and everyone else is in jeans. Someone comments about how lovely you look.

+ **Automatic negative thought:** "He's just saying that to be nice. He feels sorry for me because I look so foolish."

+ **Substitute:** "I look great in this dress and I'm going to have a fun evening!"

If some of the examples above sound familiar, you are not alone. Negative thinking patterns are traps that we all fall into at one time or another. As with many of the life-changing brain makeovers in this program, learning to identify these automatic negative thoughts and substituting them with positive, rational ones will take time and practice. If you have trouble doing this on your own or find yourself slipping back into old thinking patterns, you might want to work with a professional certified therapist who will help steer you away from these self-defeating neural pathways and offer new and better roads on which your mind can travel. The payoff is so tremendous that it is well worth the effort.

The ability to control your thoughts will allow you to gain control over your mental capabilities, your body, and your life. You can apply these skills to overcome weight problems, depression, phobias, bad habits—whatever you want to change in your life. By practicing these techniques and changing your mind-set, you will feel calmer, more confident, and joyful. People will be naturally drawn to you. So you might find that your social life will also improve. Remember, emotions are contagious, so why not spread a little happiness? As Mother Teresa said, "Let no one ever come to you without leaving better and happier."

Diane's Story

Diane, a thirty-two-year-old marketing executive, loved her job. Her colleagues respected her creativity and her ability to come up with innovative ideas. They encouraged her to apply for a more senior position where she could be instrumental in moving the company forward. She truly wanted to go for it, but the job required giving presentations, which she knew she could *never* do. Just the thought of standing up in front of a group of people sent her heart racing.

A colleague suggested that she try seeing a cognitive behavioral therapist to overcome her fear of public speaking. Having little faith that anything could help, she made an appointment anyway. On the first day, the therapist asked her to write down her feelings and thoughts when she imagined herself speaking in front of a crowd. Her laundry list included: "I'd freeze and forget what to say"; "Everyone will think I'm stupid"; "I'd make mistakes"; and "Everyone would laugh at me."

The therapist then showed Diane how to do the Relaxation Response. She was also taught to closely monitor the emotions that accompanied her thoughts. Before long, Diane discovered that when she was anxious, she was thinking anxious thoughts. When she felt insecure, she was focusing on her shortcomings. Understanding that her feelings were a product of her thoughts was a powerful revelation.

In subsequent sessions, she and her therapist went through each negative thought on her original list. Diane began to see that every one of them was a negative automatic thought that she could dismantle by using logic and replacing it with a positive thought. For example "I'd freeze and forget what to say" was replaced by "I'll be well prepared with notes that I can look at if I get stuck."

She learned to identify common types of negative thinking and realized that "Everyone will think I'm stupid" was simply untrue. Her therapist called this an "irrational thought." After all, her colleagues wouldn't encourage her to apply for the job if she wasn't clever enough to handle it. Diane also learned to watch out for thoughts that contained words such as *always*, *never*, *every*, *no one*, and *everyone*—telltale signs of all-or-nothing thinking. And she realized that her previous worry that "I'd make a mistake" was a ridiculous thing to fret about. We all make mistakes. And if we do, the world won't end. Isn't that how we learn?

During the next six weeks, Diane experienced a new sense of calm and focus. She was aware of what she was thinking and consequently feeling throughout the day. Whenever she started to feel stressed, she could calm herself with the Relaxation Response. If a negative thought popped into her head, she would immediately replace it with a positive one. Diane learned how to gain mastery over her mind. So after she was promoted to her dream job and the time came for her to give her first speech, she was ready—and it went without a hitch!

GET A MIND-LIFT

In addition to using the techniques above, there are other ways to enhance your mind-set and lift your spirit. Select a few from the suggestions below. Try them all or come up with some other ideas of your own.

✦ **Move it!** We devoted an entire step to the health benefits of movement, and studies show that regular aerobic exercise is also the perfect antidote for anxiety and stress. Remember the "fight or flight" response? When we feel stressed our body is prepared to move. Exercise releases that nervous energy and puts our mind and body back on an even keel. A quick fix when you're feeling anxious is to run up the stairs or do ten to fifteen wall push-ups. Both these quick pick-me-ups can be done just about anywhere. (Trust me: I've even done wall push-ups in the ladies' room!)

In addition, physical exercise has been found to be as effective as antidepressant medications. The latest research suggests that not only does it lift depression and treat anxiety, but it also appears to prevent it. Scientists believe that this has to do with the growth of new brain cells that occurs with aerobic activity.

✦ **Laugh it up!** Just about everyone feels better after a good laugh. The reason, studies show, is that laughter is good for our health. It reduces the level of the stress hormone cortisol and improves mood through the release of endorphins. The physical act of laughter is comparable to mild aerobic exercise and may elevate mood and decrease stress through increased blood flow to the brain. So try to spend time with people who like to chuckle. You might want to try Laughter Yoga, which was the brainchild of a physician in India. It's based on the fact that laughing is an excellent stress reliever, and it combines traditional yoga with laughter. You can also hit the comedy clubs, go to funny movies (comedies are even more fun when there is a roomful of people laughing together), watch your favorite show on Comedy Central, or read cartoons. An added benefit is that people who smile and laugh are perceived as being more attractive than those who don't.

✦ **Music therapy.** In his book *Musicophilia*, Dr. Oliver Sacks writes about the power of music, which, he says, can "move us to the heights or depths of emotion." Music therapy is increasingly being used in medical settings, from soothing premature infants in neonatal intensive care units to treating depression and triggering memory retrieval in patients with Alzheimer's. Singing has also been found to relieve stress, especially upbeat music that puts people in a good mood. So download some uplifting iTunes on your MP3, join a choir, go with friends to a karaoke bar, or sing in the shower and bathe your brain in your favorite melodies.

✦ **Memorize poetry or lyrics.** Not only is this an excellent memory exercise, but it is also downright therapeutic. Reciting words that resonate with you personally is a powerful way to buoy your spirits or strengthen your resolve. Compile your own personal mental library of inspiring poems or song lyrics that will send your soul soaring. Visit your local library or go to www.poets.org or www.songlyrics.com.

✦ **Make furry friends.** Studies have shown that pets improve our moods and relieve stress, which is why pet therapy is so widely used in nursing homes, hospitals, and special needs schools to reduce loneliness, anger, and depression. Erika Friedman, an expert in pet therapy research, found that cardiac patient survival rates were higher for those who owned pets, and that elderly people with pets made fewer visits to the doctor's office. When research subjects played with their pets, they showed a significant decrease in their resting heart rate and blood pressure, as well as positive mood changes. The unconditional love we receive from our furry friends is yet another reason to adopt a pet. (My cat, Leon, can attest to that!)

✦ **Commune with Mother Nature.** Our lives can be so frantic that we forget to pause to listen to the birds singing, the patter of rain, or the stirrings of branches in the wind. According to a University of Michigan study, people who strolled through a wooded park for fifty minutes significantly improved their performance on an attention test, while the scores of people who walked on noisy city streets prior to testing stayed the same. The relaxing atmosphere of nature gives your prefrontal cortex—the area of your brain that helps you focus—an opportunity to recharge. Whenever possible, spend time outdoors, take the scenic route home, stop to watch a sunset, and gaze at the stars. If you can't go outside, open your curtains and windows and let the sunshine and fresh air in.

✦ **Om sweet om.** Yoga prepares the mind for meditation and is one of the best ways to achieve mindfulness. It evokes the Relaxation Response through chanting, meditation, and repetitive movement. According to a study by Sara Lazar, a Harvard neuroscientist at the Benson-Henry Institute for Mind Body Medicine at Massachusetts General Hospital, meditation increases the thickness of various cortical regions and could offset age-related cortical thinning. There are many different types of yoga available today, from gentle and healing light meditation, to advanced Vinyasa, Hatha, and Bikram (hot yoga), which is done in a room heated to a minimum of 105 degrees. Pick one that fits your personality and fitness level.

✦ **Massage your mind.** Massage, which involves pressing, rubbing, and manipulating the muscles, tendons, and ligaments, is used to relieve stress, manage anxiety, reduce stiffness, and alleviate pain caused by sports injuries. It can also help control blood pressure. A good massage can feel like thirty to sixty minutes of bliss. Another way to soothe your nerves and toot-sies is to go for a pedicure, which usually includes a hot foot soak and a five-minute foot massage. Practice the RR while you indulge in these treatments for a beautifying mind boost.

✦ **Put your energy where your heart is.** Volunteer for a char-ity or cause that you believe in. Altruism and volunteerism are associated with well-being, happiness, health, and longevity. The humanitarian and brain rewards are limitless!

✦ **Friends and family plan.** The camaraderie of friends and family is a wonderful way to calm our spirits and to keep our emotional sails buoyed. In fact cultures that understand the importance of family ties tend to experience the greatest hap-piness and longevity. The Jack and Jill Late Stage Cancer Foun-dation, which provides all-expense-paid vacations for people who can't afford them, has helped many a family enjoy precious time together knowing that the person who is ill might not be around for graduations, wedding ceremonies, and grandkids. Don't wait for devastating news to cherish the memories you create spending time with your friends and loved ones.

GET READY FOR THE SMART DIET

Now that you have learned how to relax and control your negative thoughts, you can be open to the idea of mindful eating. The Smart Diet involves making intelligent choices when it comes to what you put inside your body and rethinking some of your old unhealthy eating habits. *Bon appétit!*

The Smart Diet

*If you are what you eat and you don't know what
you're eating, do you know who you are?*
—CLAUDE FISCHLER, FRENCH SOCIOLOGIST

DON'T DIET, LIVE IT!

There is no question that what we put in our body directly affects
how our brain operates and how we look and feel on the outside. But
Step six of your beauty/brain makeover is *not* about dieting (the
verb), which almost always involves deprivation. It's about spicing up
your life by eating the Smart Diet, which means heartily indulging in
nutritious foods and a variety of cuisines that will give your brain
and body the most bang for their buck. It's about why eating should
be one of our greatest pleasures and should never be done mind-
lessly. Like the Relaxation Response, eating is another way to get in
touch with our senses and the world around us. I will ask you to em-
ploy what I call "mindful eating" so you can savor every morsel and
sip that you take. I also suggest that you share your meals with family
and friends as much as possible as a way to improve your life as well
as your brain.

And while we know that obesity is bad for us, don't beat yourself up over the number on the scale. If your life constantly revolves around what you eat, I say don't diet, live it! The stress of constant yo-yo dieting is counterproductive to your brain and body, so concentrate instead on plentiful consumption of foods that are both delicious and good for you. The reason why those who live near the Mediterranean tend to live longer and have lower rates of obesity than Americans may have has as much to do with their slower-paced, family-friendly lifestyle and attitudes toward food as it does with their diet.

Mediterranean Thinking

Studies have shown a Mediterranean diet is associated with a reduced risk of developing memory difficulties and Alzheimer's disease. A 2004 Greek study by Theodora Psaltopoulou published in the *Journal of Nutrition* found that intakes of olive oil, vegetables, and fish were associated with lower blood pressure, while cereals, meat, and alcohol were associated with higher blood pressure.

RESET YOUR MIND BEFORE YOU SET YOUR TABLE

Before we begin our Smart Diet, I want you to adopt the proper mealtime mind-set. Our goal is to replace all the negative thoughts you have about food and body image with positive, self-affirming ones. Keep in mind that healthy attitudes toward food and body image will naturally result in a healthy weight in the long run. The first step involves pausing to take pleasure in our food. Consider this passage from Elizabeth Gilbert's wonderful book *Eat Pray Love*:

> I walked home to my apartment and soft boiled a pair of fresh brown eggs for my lunch. I peeled the eggs and arranged them on a plate beside the seven stalks of asparagus (which were so slim and snappy they didn't need to be cooked at all). I put some olives on the plate, too, and the four knobs of goat cheese I'd picked up yesterday from the *formaggeria* down the street, and two slices of pink, oily salmon. For dessert—a lovely peach . . . still warm from the Roman sunlight. For the longest time I couldn't even touch this food because it was such a masterpiece of lunch, a true expression of the art of making something out of nothing. Finally, when I had fully absorbed the prettiness of my meal, I went and sat in a patch of sunbeam on my clean wooden floor and ate every bite of it, with my fingers. . . . Happiness inhabited my every molecule.

As Gilbert so delightfully described, when we are mindful of what we eat, not only do we enjoy it more, but it is also more satisfying because it nourishes both our body and our soul. Mindful eating will fill you up in ways that *mindless* grazing never will. Here are some other suggestions for savoring your meals:

✦ **Get fresh.** Whether you're at a restaurant or grocery store, always choose the freshest and most unadulterated fruits, vegetables, and other foods so you can truly savor nature's bounty. Local foods are better than those that have traveled long distances because nutrient levels begin to decline as soon as food is harvested. The fresher it is, the better it will taste.

✦ **Prepare with love.** Take time to arrange your food so that it looks attractive—this includes takeout. Use your prettiest dishes and goblets, even if it's just you, or the family. Who could be more important? Garnish with fresh herbs, citrus, and relishes to embellish the "presentation." Food that looks good is more satisfying.

✦ **Ambiance is everything.** Eating in a beautiful, relaxed setting enhances the taste of our food. So enjoy your lunch break at a local park, request the window seat at your favorite restaurant, and add a floral arrangement or candlelight when you dine at home. In my husband's family, candles were lit at every meal, including breakfast. We've continued this tradition at our evening meal, which radiates a calming atmosphere over our table.

✦ **Share with others.** Mealtime is a wonderful time to share with friends and family. Remember that socializing with others is great for your brain. Numerous studies show that having regular family meals is related to better nutritional intake and decreases the risk of eating disorders and substance abuse in children. I suspect the same holds true for adults!

✦ **Give thanks.** One of my favorite family traditions is to join hands with those around our table and pause to give thanks. Even if you're alone, filling your heart with gratitude is the perfect way to set your mind at the start of every meal.

Don't Eat for Love

Do you love to eat, or do you eat for love? When we are sad, depressed, and lonely, or suffering from PMS, we might reach for that pint of ice cream or plate of pasta in order to soothe our sorry selves. Try to find other ways to elevate your mood, such as going for a walk or run, reading a good book, or watching a comedy. If your depression and comfort food habit are chronic, talk to your doctor.

THE BEAUTY OF THE SMART DIET

The Smart Diet allows you to look, think, and perform at the top of your game because your brain and body are getting the nutrients they need to function at their very best. It involves making smart choices and understanding that what you eat *and* what you don't eat make a difference both in the short term and in the long run. The Smart Diet explains how the foods you eat affect not only the structure and function of your body but *also* your brain. And as you know, the sharper your brain, the better you will look and feel. I'm sure you've heard the saying "You are what you eat." I have added my own personal mantra to that one, which is: "You *think* what you eat."

When we eat foods that are filled with sugar, artery-clogging fats, and artificial additives we are altering our brain chemistry. In the short term this can affect our mood and concentration. In the long term, it invites the Brain Beauty Burglars (obesity, high blood pressure, diabetes, and high cholesterol) to rob us of our intellectual power and beauty.

Women who skip meals or go on crash diets are depriving their brain and their body of proper nutrition. As a result, they often get that sallow look and feel grouchy. They might also feel dizzy and mentally fatigued. Have you ever wondered why you're more likely to be irritable and have difficulty focusing when you're dieting? What we eat directly affects our mood and our ability to concentrate. Again, it all has to do with altering our brain chemistry. Despite what many women think, crash and yo-yo dieting take a toll on your appearance by depleting your body of beautifying nutrients and inducing muscle loss. And one of the keys to aging well is to maintain our muscle mass, which keeps us strong and gives our body definition.

Adopting the Smart Diet beautifies your brain and your body. It is rich in Smart Fats such as omega-3 fatty acids that not only boost your brain power but also naturally lubricate your skin, making it look smoother and more youthful. It promotes strong teeth and bones by supplying ample sources of calcium and other minerals necessary for bone health. This is especially important for older women who are at risk of osteoporosis (bone thinning). The Smart Diet also contains nutritious sources of protein, a necessary building block for strong muscles, healthy hair, and sturdy nails.

Remember what I said about how aging begins within our cells? The Smart Diet, which is rich in phytonutrients (more about this later), has antiaging properties that will keep your cells flourishing and your arteries open—promoting better blood flow throughout your body. Not only your brain but also your skin and hair follicles thrive on nourishing and oxygenated blood flow.

The Smart Diet also encourages you to indulge in a variety of foods that are naturally low in calories and prevent your blood sugar from spiking, both of which have antiaging effects. The diet keeps hormone levels such as insulin low, which promotes natural weight loss. High insulin levels cause us to gain weight, especially in our abdomen. This creates a health risk and increases the chronic inflammation that further ages our cells. In short, by adopting the Smart Diet you will improve not only your overall health, but you will also start to see a beautiful transformation that will take place from the inside and out.

SMART CARBS

Like cholesterol, there are "good" carbohydrates and "bad" ones. Most nutrition experts agree that plants are at the top of the "intelligent" food chain. In fact pretty much all vegetables, fruits, legumes, and whole grains are what I call Smart Carbs. It all has to do with how quickly our blood sugar rises after eating carbohydrates. Smart Carbs cause a slow rise in blood sugar. You see, all carbs are broken down into sugar, which is absorbed into our bloodstream. The *slower* our blood sugar rises after eating, the *better*. This is because high blood sugar levels trigger a rise in insulin levels, both of which take a toll on our cells and make us age faster.

By consuming Smart Carbs, which release their sugar content slowly, your blood sugar and insulin levels stay in a low, healthy range. Natural, unprocessed foods such as vegetables, fruits, and whole grains contain fiber, which naturally slows the absorption of sugar, so they are the best sources of carbohydrates for your body.

Conversely, when we regularly eat Bad Carbs, such as sweets and processed foods that are stripped of their natural fiber, our blood sugar rises rapidly. The faster our blood sugar rises, the bigger the insulin spike. High glucose and insulin spikes eventually wreak havoc on both your body and your brain. They negatively impact our brain cells, particularly those in the vital hippocampus memory center. Bad Carbs promote weight gain (especially in the abdomen), inflammation, and increased LDL (the bad cholesterol), which clogs blood vessels. Regularly consuming Bad Carbs also increases your risk of developing prediabetes and diabetes, those notorious Brain Beauty Burglars.

Keeping your blood sugar and insulin levels on an even keel by eating Smart Carbs will promote better brain function, reduce your risk of Alzheimer's and stroke, and naturally trim your waistline. In the following section, I'll tell you which carbs to avoid and which ones are loaded with beautifying nutrients and compounds that help keep you looking younger and more vibrant.

DON'T RUN WITH THE BAD CARB CROWD

A good way to avoid falling in with the Bad Carb crowd is to steer clear of refined foods, processed foods, and those with added sugar such as white breads, sweetened cereals, cookies, crackers, chips, candy, white potatoes, and white rice. (Although white rice and white potatoes are natural foods, their sugars are quickly absorbed into the bloodstream and are therefore not recommended.)

Identifying Bad Carbs can be tricky. The first clue that a food may be a Bad Carb is that it comes in a package or a wrapper. A laundry list of ingredients, especially with words that are hard to pronounce and sound like something found in a chemistry lab, is a good indicator that it is a highly processed food and contains Bad Carbs.

Be sure to read labels and watch out for "flour." Unless the first ingredient contains the words *whole*, such as *whole* grain, *whole* wheat, or *whole* meal, it's most likely a Bad Carb. For example, "wheat flour" is no better than white flour. It will say "whole grain wheat flour" or "whole wheat flour" if it truly meets whole grain criteria. And don't be fooled by the color of breads and other flour-containing products such as chips and crackers. Manufacturers often add molasses or coloring to darken them and make them appear more wholesome.

Most important, watch out for added sugar. Even honey, brown sugar, and organic sugarcane, which sound somewhat wholesome, will nonetheless send your blood sugar soaring. A good rule of thumb is to avoid products that list sugar (or one of its aliases) in the first three ingredients. Be aware that manufacturers disguise sugar by using a variety of names, such as cane juice, corn sweetener, beet sugar, fruit juice concentrate, corn syrup, barley malt, fructose, sucrose, and our old friend glucose. These stealthy sugars, which you will find in many processed foods and sodas, cause your blood sugar and insulin levels to spike, leading to weight gain, inflammation, clogged arteries, and an unhealthy brain and body.

FABULOUS PHYTONUTRIENTS

In addition to keeping our blood sugar and insulin levels low, Smart Carbs are rich in "phytonutrients"—nature's most powerful beautifying agents. *Phytonutrient* is the umbrella term for all the chemical compounds found in plants or fruits, vegetables, legumes, grains, and grasses that are beneficial to humans and other living things. *Phyto* means "plant," and of course *nutrients* speaks for itself. Antioxidants and vitamins are just two kinds of phytonutrient—there are many others that haven't even been explored yet.

In fact phytonutrients found in different types of plants across the globe have antioxidant, anti-inflammatory, antiviral, antibacterial, immune-boosting, and cellular-repairing properties. Eating a diet rich in fruits, vegetables, legumes, and whole grains (aka Smart Carbs) ensures that you will reap the benefits that nature has to offer. Even a variety of supplements can't possibly supply the thousands of phytonutrients that are present in plants. For example, a simple orange is estimated to contain more than 170 phytonutrients, including flavanones and polyphenols, which protect our skin and have antiaging properties.

Natural foods also supply nutrients in the perfect dosage. Our bodies have evolved to absorb tiny concentrations of these phytonutrients found in plants, not the megadoses found in supplements. In fact, super-high doses of some phytonutrients, as found in supplements, may become "pro-oxidants," which can promote cellular dysfunction and destruction.

Unlike supplements, plant nutrients come in just the right combinations. Spinach, for example, is an excellent source of iron and vitamin C, and the presence of vitamin C boosts our ability to absorb iron. It is impossible to achieve this perfect synergy when taking supplements—yet another reason why it's best to eat whole foods. Eating a wide variety of Smart Carbs in the form of fruits, vegetables, and whole grains will ensure that you get all the nutrients you need to stay vibrant and beautiful.

BE COLORFUL

The more colorful your meals, the better they are for you. I'm not talking about food coloring, of course, but adding something green, red, yellow, purple, blue, and orange to your meals. Why are colors so important? Phytonutrients produce the distinctive bright colors in fruits and vegetables. These essential nutrients assist in thousands of cell processes throughout our brain and body. Phytonutrients that have antioxidant properties protect your brain and your body from toxic free radicals. Free radicals, a product of cell metabolism, cause cellular destruction and injury. They are believed to play a role in aging as well as many neurodegenerative diseases, including Alzheimer's.

In addition to antioxidant properties, phytonutrients protect our tissues from cancer, decrease inflammation, enhance immune function, and have age-defying properties that keep our cells young. And as you now know, if your cells are healthy, you will radiate that wholesome glow. Eating a variety of colors enables your brain and body to get the nutrients they need to function at their best, because similar protective compounds often display similar hues. For example, the deep orange color of sweet potatoes and carrots comes from antiaging phytonutrients that help protect our skin against sun damage, wrinkles, redness, and skin cancer. So in order to reap the beautiful bounty that nature offers, be sure to eat a little from each color family. Remember, it takes a rainbow to make a nourishing meal, and every color in the palette brings something different to the table.

◆ **The green family.** Eating your greens is one of the most important dietary steps you can take for your brain. A long-range Harvard Medical School study of more than thirteen thousand aging women found that those who frequently ate green leafy vegetables lowered their mental age in terms of performance by one to two years, compared to those who did not. Dark green leafy vegetables are rich in the phytonutrients we talked about, and studies show that they can prevent macular degeneration and cataracts, which can lead to blindness. The green family includes spinach, kale, beet greens, collards, green beans, artichokes, green peppers, okra, leeks, edamame, avocados, green apples, kiwi, and honeydew. Other green cruciferous vegetables known for their cancer-fighting elements are broccoli, brussels sprouts, cabbage, kale, and bok choy. Aim for at least one serving per day. Kermit notwithstanding, it is very easy to be green.

✦ **The blue/purple family.** Some of the most powerful antioxidant foods that are great for your brain and vision are in the blue/purple family. Aging rats whose diets were supplemented by antioxidant-rich blueberries, for example, were found to be more curious and have better memories than those that were not. Other blue/purple family members include blackberries, raspberries, black currants, grapes/raisins, plums/prunes, pomegranates, eggplant, purple cabbage, purple peppers, and black beans.

✦ **The red family.** The red foods are very rich in phytonutrients with antioxidant effects. In fact, eight of the top twenty antioxidant foods ranked by the USDA are red. These include small red beans, red kidney beans, cranberries, strawberries, red delicious apples, sweet cherries, and gala apples. Tomatoes and tomato products are an important component of this family. Unlike most fruits and vegetables, which lose nutrients when cooked, the cancer-fighting benefits in tomatoes increases with cooking. Other foods in this family include red bell peppers, red chili peppers, radishes, red onions, beets, radicchio, currants, red grapefruit, guava, papaya, watermelon, rhubarb, and red pears.

✦ **The orange family.** Brighten up your plate and brain with orange foods. Many of the orange foods can be cold stored. If you grocery shop once a week, stock up on these to use later on. Examples include carrots, squash, sweet potatoes, orange bell peppers, pumpkin, oranges, tangerines, peaches, nectarines, mangoes, apricots, cantaloupe, papaya, and persimmon.

Phytonutrients in the orange family protect our skin from sun damage and wrinkles.

✦ **The yellow family.** Many of the fruits and vegetables in this group have a milder taste and can be a great choice for children who are picky eaters. Both yellow and orange foods are high in beta- and alpha-carotene, which the body converts into vitamin A. This vitamin is important for healthy skin, nails, and hair. Try yellow squash, yellow wax beans, corn, yellow bell peppers, pineapple, bananas, yellow pears, golden delicious apples, and grapefruit.

✦ **The white/tan family.** This group makes up for its lack of color with a variety of nutrients that maintain healthy immune systems and appear to improve memory. A study by Saida Haider in the *Journal of Medicinal Food* showed how rats that were fed fresh garlic regularly performed better on memory tests. So be sure to include garlic, onions, mushrooms, turnips, cauliflower, garbanzo beans, bananas, dates, figs, and brown pears in your diet.

Going Organic

Organic produce is touted as having more antioxidants than conventionally grown produce, but this is difficult to confirm, given that the quality of the soil and weather are such big factors. There have been some studies showing higher levels of antioxidant activity in organically grown blueberries, carrots, and tomatoes, but other studies show no significant difference. Perhaps most important when buying produce is how fresh and vibrant it appears. A deep red tomato will have more nutrients and taste better than one that looks anemic. It is also worth considering how far the food has traveled since being harvested. Produce begins losing nutrients once it is harvested. Locally grown produce has an advantage in this regard, so stop by the farmer's market or start your own organic garden.

The bigger issue when choosing between organic and conventionally grown produce is pesticide exposure. Pesticides such as organophosphates are neurotoxins that are specifically designed to attack the central nervous system of pests. While we know the detrimental effects on humans from poisoning by acute high-level exposure, the effects of chronic low-level exposure are still unknown. Multiple studies show a link between pesticide exposure and an increased risk of Parkinson's disease, a progressive neurological disorder that causes degeneration of neurons in the region of the brain that controls movement. Studies of other neurodegenerative diseases such as Alzheimer's disease are limited. However, it seems wise to limit your consumption of pesticides by buying organic foods, especially for produce where you don't peel the skin, such as apples, peaches, berries, grapes, and lettuce.

And because buying organic can be costly, you might want to purchase frozen organic fruits and vegetables, which are less expensive and retain much of their nutrients. I find frozen organic berries and other seasonal produce a convenient way to enjoy these nutritious foods throughout the year. Frozen fruits and vegetables also tide me over between weekly grocery shopping trips when I run low on fresh produce. For limited budgets, don't spend valuable food dollars on organic ingredients in processed foods, since processing changes the chemical composition of foods and may limit the benefits. Not to mention, you're best off avoiding processed foods.

BRILLIANT BRAIN FATS

Nearly 60 percent of the human brain is composed of fat or "lipids." The fats you consume literally become the buildings blocks for your brain. This is why choosing the best fats is one of the most important dietary decisions you can make to keep your brain vibrant and beautiful. As you now know, the right balance of healthy fats keeps blood vessels free of plaque, ensuring good blood flow to the brain. Unhealthy fats not only clog the arteries that nourish the brain but also negatively influence mood and impair communication among brain cells.

The most important miracle foods for your brain are those rich in omega-3 fatty acids such as those found in fatty fish, and flaxseed oil (see Smart Fats on page 181). These Smart Fats are absolutely vital for a healthy brain. Omega 3s are also known as "essential fatty acids" because our body can't make them. And nothing could be more "essential" than ensuring that our brain has an adequate supply of these super nutrients by making smart dietary choices. Numerous studies have linked dietary omega-3 intake to improved blood flow, increased brain cell growth, improved mood, and better memory. Diets high in omega-3s are also associated with lower rates of Alzheimer's disease.

Omega-3s appear to protect arteries from plaque buildup, and studies suggest that diets high in omega-3s enhance learning and memory and decrease the risk of stroke and dementia. They also appear to be important in making new neurons in the hippocampus; and getting an adequate amount of omega-3 is vital for fetal brain development. I can't overemphasize how important it is to get enough omega-3s in your diet, and I will explain how you can do this later on. But first you need to get the skinny on fats.

THE SKINNY ON FATS

Understanding nutritional fats can be confusing, so let me try to simplify the chemistry to help you make smart choices for your brain. There are two main types of fats: *unsaturated* and *saturated*. Fats are made up of carbon, oxygen, and hydrogen and are named by how much hydrogen they can carry. Unsaturated fats have room for more hydrogen, while saturated fats are maxed out on hydrogen and can't add any more, hence the term *saturated*. Unsaturated fats turn to liquid at room temperature and are great for your brain, while saturated fats are solid at room temperature and are bad for your brain.

Research shows that unsaturated fats (which include omega-3s) improve the flexibility of neuronal membranes, which in essence could make you smarter. This is why I call these Smart Fats. And because saturated fats make neuronal membranes less fluid, I will refer to them as Inflexible Fats, which highlights the fact that consuming these fats can lead to mental inflexibility—not a flattering image.

Smart (Unsaturated) Fats

Unsaturated (Smart) fats are derived from nuts, seeds, vegetables, and fish. There are two main types of unsaturated fats: monounsaturated and polyunsaturated. Examples of monounsaturated fats are olive and canola oil. Polyunsaturated fats include our beloved omega-3s as well as omega-6s. The best source of omega-3s is fatty fish, but they can also be found in flaxseed oil and walnuts. Other less potent sources of omega-3s include pumpkin seeds, soy beans, tofu, pecans, and fortified eggs. Omega-6s are found in vegetable oils such as corn and safflower.

While both omega-3s and omega-6s are important for our brain function, the ratio of these two dietary fats is extremely important. The ideal ratio of omega-6 to omega-3 is three to one. That is, we should get three times as much omega-6 as omega-3. Unfortunately the average American diet is estimated to have a ratio of twenty to one, which is an extremely unhealthy balance for the brain. This means we're getting way too much omega-6 and not nearly enough omega-3. Our overconsumption of vegetable oils containing omega-6, which are used in processed foods, is largely to blame, as is the fact that our diets are lacking in healthy fats. Eating fish will improve your ratio, as fish oil has *seven* times as much omega-3 as omega-6. The bottom line for brain-boosting Smart Fats is to substitute olive oil or canola oil for vegetable oil when cooking and to eat more foods that are rich in omega-3s.

Smart Fat Roundup

✦ Eat fatty fish at least twice a week for their potent omega-3s: DHA and EPA (see page 190 for examples). Fatty fish offers the best source of omega-3s for your brain, your heart, and your body. If you cannot eat fish, consider taking fish oils. Be sure to check with your doctor first.

✦ If you cannot eat fish or take fish oils, consider taking flax-seed oil, which contains the omega-3 called ALA. Unfortunately not everyone is able to convert ALA into DHA and EPA—the valuable omega-3s that are found in fish. As always, discuss with your doctor.

✦ Enjoy other less potent sources of omega-3s such as pumpkin seeds, walnuts, soybeans, tofu, pecans, and fortified eggs.

✦ Use monounsaturated oils, such as olive, peanut, sesame, and canola, in food preparation instead of corn, soy, safflower, cottonseed, or mixed vegetable oils to improve the balance of omega-3s to omega-6s.

Inflexible (Saturated) Fats

These fats are found in animal products, including whole milk, cream, butter, egg yolks, fatty meats, poultry skin, and plant products such as coconut and palm oil. While all of these fats can make your brain less flexible, trans fats are the worst. Trans fats are artificially made by treating oils with hydrogen gas, which turns them into stiff, inflexible, saturated fats. These extremely unhealthy fats go by the name "hydrogenated" or "partially hydrogenated" oils.

Manufacturers started using trans fats in processed foods because they are cheap and increase the shelf life of the product. They are found in many commercially prepared, processed, fried, and snack foods. Trans fats raise the level of your bad LDL cholesterol and lower the level of your good HDL cholesterol—a double whammy that clogs arteries throughout the brain and body. As you now know, clogged arteries impede nourishing blood flow, which in turn accelerates aging. Diets that are high in saturated fats are one of the leading causes of weight gain in Americans, and they also appear to have a negative impact on your memory. So the take-home message for inflexible fats is to avoid processed food, limit dairy to low-fat products, and eat only lean meats in small amounts.

Inflexible Fat Roundup

✦ Avoid trans fats at all costs. They are commonly found in fast foods such as fried chicken, biscuits, fried fish sandwiches,

French fries, donuts, muffins, crackers, cookies, cake, icing, pie, microwave popcorn, canned biscuits, and instant latte coffee beverages.

✦ Read labels on packaged foods and stay away from any products with the words *partially hydrogenated* or *hydrogenated*, which means a trans fat.

✦ Steer clear of margarine and other products that contain coconut and palm kernel oil, which are high in saturated fats.

✦ It's best to avoid red meat, but if you do eat it, purchase lean cuts, trim excess fat, and limit intake. Quality also matters. Grass-fed or pasture-raised meat is the healthiest beef you can buy.

✦ For poultry, avoid skin and trim excess fat. Limit to twice a week. Again, quality matters, and free range is best.

✦ For dairy, avoid or limit cream, whole milk, and butter. Low-fat dairy is best.

THE POWER OF PROTEIN

Did you know that your muscles, skin, and hair are all made of protein? Not surprisingly, eating the right kinds of protein will fortify your muscles, give you younger-looking skin, stronger nails, and shinier, healthier hair. But that's not all: Protein, which is made up of amino acids, is also in many of our bodies' important chemicals, including neurotransmitters, hormones, and enzymes. Our body uses twenty amino acids to manufacture the more than 100,000 proteins required for structure, function, and regulation of our tissues and organs. Our body can make eleven of these twenty amino acids. The other nine must come from our diet and are called "essential amino acids." Fish, poultry, eggs, meat, milk, and cheese provide all the essential amino acids we need. Proteins that come from plants, including legumes, grains, and vegetables, tend to be limited in essential amino acids. However vegetarians can get all the essential amino acids as long as they maintain a reasonably varied diet.

According to the Centers for Disease Control and Prevention, the average female needs 46 grams of protein a day. A three-ounce serving of fish, four ounces of soybeans, and one cup of low-fat yogurt meet this requirement. Considering all the things our body uses protein for, it's not that much. This is because our body recycles protein. In fact most of us get far more protein than we need. There are circumstances, however, when we do need more protein, such as during pregnancy, lactation, healing from trauma or illness, and with aggressive endurance training such as preparing for a marathon. In these cases, nutritional counseling can be helpful.

So what are the best sources of protein? A Smart Diet should contain protein that comes primarily from fish and plant vegetable sources. This is because you need to consider what else comes with the protein. Fish is an excellent source of protein and also provides the Smart Fats that can't be beat. Plant sources such as beans, whole grains, and nuts are also an excellent choice, offering healthy fiber and phytonutrients. Low-fat dairy products offer all the essential amino acids and are a good source of calcium. Poultry is a good choice, provided the skin and excess fat are removed, but it's best to limit it to twice a week. Like poultry, eggs are a good source of protein and other nutrients, but due to the animal fat in the yolk, limit them to twice a week. If I can't convince you to give up red meat, with its saturated inflexible fats, stick with the leanest cuts and reserve it for special occasions only.

Smart Diet Protein Roundup

Here are some pointers to ensure you're getting enough protein and the best sources for your brain, body, skin, hair, and nails.

✦ Limit red meat and opt instead for fish, seafood, or plant sources, including legumes, nuts, seeds, and whole grains. Low-fat dairy with its bone-building calcium is also a good choice, as is lean poultry. Limit eggs to twice a week due to the animal fat in the yolk.

✦ Aim for 46 grams of protein per day.

✦ Older women often don't consume enough protein. Studies show that when elderly people don't get enough protein they are more apt to break a hip or are more likely to suffer poor medical outcomes.

✦ Special circumstances when we need more protein include pregnancy, lactation, healing from trauma or illness, and during aggressive endurance training

SMART DIET BRAIN BEAUTY BOOSTERS

Now that you understand the major food groups that make up the Smart Diet, here is a list of the essential foods that will keep your brain, body, skin, nails, and hair beautiful.

✦ **Fish.** When it comes to brain boosters, fish is the best. It truly is brain food. No other food provides the generous amounts of DHA and EPA omega-3 fatty acids that are linked to better blood flow, increased growth of brain cells, improved mood, lower rates of depression, and better cognition. The best brain-boosting fish to choose from include cold water fatty fish such as salmon, bluefish, herring, sardines, mackerel, tuna, and trout. Wild caught is better than farm raised. Aim for at least two four-ounce servings per week. Fatty fish are also the best beauty food around and will beautify your skin, hair, and nails. They are an excellent source of protein—the building blocks for healthy skin, hair, and nails. Fish oils naturally lubricate our skin from the inside out, making it smooth and supple, and prevent our hair and nails from becoming dry and brittle.

✦ **Fruits and veggies.** Filling your plate with a variety of colorful fruits and vegetables will ensure that your brain and body receive all the phytonutrients they need to stay beautiful. Fruits and veggies are rich in potassium, magnesium, and calcium, and have the added benefit of lowering blood pressure, which your brain will love. And they also provide fiber, which helps lower cholesterol. Getting lots of plant foods into your diet is key to a healthy brain. Aim for four to six half-cup servings of fruit and five to seven half-cup servings of veggies every day. I know it seems like a lot—but it's easier to do than you might think.

Broaden your palate and explore Mother Nature's bounty by trying new fruits and veggies the next time you're out to eat. Be more adventuresome when you're at the market and go for that lovely produce that you normally pass by. Why not try blood oranges, tangerines, tangelos, or clementines instead of the "ordinary" orange? Don't forget that these Smart Carbs are loaded with antiaging phytonutrients and will keep your sugar and insulin levels low, which also promotes weight loss. Making fruits and veggies a priority at every meal will enhance your brain and your beauty, and slim your waistline.

✦ **Legumes.** This special class of nutritious vegetables, which includes beans, peas, and lentils, deserves special attention. And yes, they count when you tally your veggie servings per day! Legumes are high in protein and fiber and low in fat—the nutritional holy trinity. They have been a staple for people around the world for thousands of years.

Cheaper than meat and lower in fat, legumes are an important part of your Smart Diet. A one-pound bag of dried beans costs only a few dollars and contains enough for many meals. When you cook at home, you have the added bonus of being able to control the amount of salt needed, as canned beans can be high in sodium. There's a colorful variety to choose from: kidney beans, black beans, lima beans, black-eyed peas, edamame, chickpeas, Anasazi, fava, and lentils—which come in brown, green, red, orange, white, and black!

As you might guess from their colors, they also offer an array of phytonutrients. Legumes are an excellent source of iron, biotin, and zinc, which are important for healthy hair. Iron deficiency is a common cause of female hair loss. So keep your locks luscious by making legumes an integral part of your Smart Diet.

✦ **Whole grains.** Whole grains, which come in all shapes and sizes—from large kernel popcorn to tiny quinoa seeds—should be an essential part of any Smart Diet. Whole grains are a good source of complex carbohydrates as well as various vitamins and minerals, and are naturally low in fat. They're also an excellent source of fiber. Choose whole grain breads, pastas, and cereals rather than their refined counterparts. If in doubt, check the label.

The word *whole* followed by the type of grain should be among the first items in the ingredients list. There is a wide assortment of whole grains waiting for you to try, including barley, oats, farro, buckwheat, wild rice, bulgur, millet, smelt, and brown rice.

✦ **Poultry.** Lean meats such as poultry are a good choice, provided the excess fat is removed. Chicken is a significant source of protein, niacin, B6, B12, vitamin D, iron, and zinc. Ounce for ounce, skinless chicken is one of the lowest-fat meats around, and white breast meat is lower in fat than dark meat. Additionally, a good portion of the fat it does have is unsaturated—the good kind of fat. Prepared the right way, chicken is low in calories and cholesterol. Turkey is another good source of lean protein. A three-ounce serving of boneless, skinless turkey breast contains 26 grams of protein, 1 gram of fat, and 0 grams of saturated fat.

✦ **Dairy.** Low-fat dairy is not only a great source of calcium and protein, but it can also help you lose those extra pounds. Numerous studies show that dairy products can play an important role in fat burning and weight loss. A study by Michael Zimmel, Ph.D., found that three daily servings of dairy products accelerated weight and body fat loss when compared to diets without dairy. His work showed that dairy sources of calcium speed up weight loss to a greater degree than calcium supplements. It is believed that the rich concentration of amino acids and other compounds in dairy products act in concert with calcium to promote weight loss. Be sure that you choose only low-fat dairy products if you want to avoid unhealthy animal fats and extra calories. If you are lactose intolerant, there are numerous alternatives to choose from. For yogurt, go with those that contain active cultures, which may have health-promoting effects.

✦ **Nuts and seeds.** Nuts and seeds are among the best plant sources of protein and healthy fats. They are also rich in phyto-nutrients, including vitamin E and selenium. If you're watching calories, limit yourself to one or two ounces daily. Mother Nature is bountiful, giving us walnuts, almonds, pecans, Brazil nuts, peanuts, cashews, pistachio, pine, hazel, and macadamia to pick from. Seeds are a nutritious way to flavor your dishes; try adding sesame, caraway, fennel, poppy, and sunflower seeds to your repertoire.

Go Fish

There is much concern about contaminants in fish such as PCBs and mercury, but the benefits still outweigh the risks as long as you follow the FDA guidelines. The same is true even for pregnant women, as studies show that fish intake is associated with better fetal brain development. But pregnant women, those in their childbearing years, and children should strictly adhere to the FDA safety guidelines. As recommendations may change over time, please visit the FDA Web site at www.fda.gov for the most up-to-date advice. Below are the current guidelines:

✦ Do not eat shark, swordfish, king mackerel, or tilefish, because they contain high levels of mercury.

✦ Eat up to twelve ounces (two average meals) a week of a variety of fish and shellfish that are lower in mercury.

✦ Five of the most commonly eaten fish that are low in mercury are shrimp, canned light tuna, salmon, pollock, and catfish.

+ Another commonly eaten fish, albacore ("white") tuna, has more mercury than canned light tuna. So when choosing your two meals of fish and shellfish, you may eat up to six ounces (one average meal) of albacore tuna per week.

+ Check local advisories about the safety of fish caught by family and friends in your local lakes, rivers, and coastal areas. If no advice is available, eat up to six ounces (one average meal) per week of fish you catch from local waters, but don't consume any other fish during that week.

+ Follow these same recommendations when feeding fish and shellfish to children, but serve smaller portions.

SPICE IT UP!

Your brain makeover is all about spicing up your life, and the same brain benefits apply when you add seasoning to your food! Many studies show that spices and herbs are rich in phytonutrients and, in particular, powerful antioxidants. Curcumin, a spice used in Indian curries, in particular, has been getting a lot of attention. It is a dietary staple in India, a country where the rate of Alzheimer's disease is among the world's lowest. This bright yellow component of turmeric and curry powder has both anti-inflammatory and antioxidant properties. In fact exciting research at Massachusetts General Hospital by Drs. Brian Bacskai and Brad Hyman found that curcumin can prevent new Alzheimer's plaques from forming and actually clear existing plaques in mice. The spice is now being studied in patients with Alzheimer's disease, so given what we now know, why not add curry dishes to your meal plans?

But don't limit the spice in your life to just curry. As I mentioned on page 178, rats that were repeatedly fed fresh garlic had increased serotonin neurotransmitter levels and improved memory function. Many other spices are known to have potent antioxidant properties, including cloves, allspice, sage, rosemary, oregano, thyme, ginger, yellow mustard seed, parsley, basil, and marjoram. There have also been several studies that show cinnamon can lower the rise in glucose and insulin, which was observed in diabetics as well as in healthy subjects. In the same way that the Smart Diet should include a variety of fruits and vegetables, it should also consist of a number of different spices and herbs. Forget the old-school saltshaker and spice up your life and your neurons!

Shake Off the Salt

Breaking the salt habit can significantly lower your blood pressure, which you now know is great for your brain. To lower blood pressure, experts recommend consuming less than 2,400 milligrams of sodium per day (about the amount in a teaspoon of salt). Those with high blood pressure should aim for 1,500 milligrams. Reading labels and avoiding salty foods can have dramatic health benefits. Never add salt before you've tasted your food. The food you get at a restaurant has already been seasoned, and I guarantee that most prepared foods you buy at the supermarket will have hidden salt and sugar. In fact most of the salt in our diet comes from processed foods and prepared meals in restaurants. If you find that you want more flavor, try using onions, garlic, pepper, lemon, lime, fresh herbs, and other spices instead. Watch out for hidden sodium in mixed seasonings and condiments. If you're the salty type, wean yourself off slowly. You'll find that once you start limiting salt for two weeks, you will be able to taste your food better. You can change your taste buds the same way you change your brain.

COFFEE, TEA, OR CAFFEINE-FREE?

For many Americans, that first cup of Joe in the morning is part of their daily ritual. Without it, we feel tired, less alert, and even experience headaches. It's no wonder that many of us are lifelong caffeine addicts, given that some of our favorite childhood soft drinks are also chock-full of caffeine (see Fizzle Out Soda on page 195). Although a cup of coffee will give us a mental boost in the short term, limiting our caffeine consumption may be a good idea in the long run.

Have you ever noticed yourself getting jittery after one too many visits to Starbucks? This is because caffeine is a stimulant that raises blood pressure and heart rate. A 2006 study in *Journal of Physiology* showed that caffeine exaggerates the stress response, which in excess can take a toll on your health and your brain. But it is often when we are under stress that we reach for that extra cup to give us a jolt, even though it actually intensifies our level of stress and makes us feel more anxious. For these reasons, it is best to limit or avoid caffeine when you feel stressed or if you suffer from anxiety or panic attacks.

Caffeine may also interfere with restorative sleep, often leading to a vicious cycle of dependency. We need that first cup in the morning to get us going and to keep going during the day, but the caffeine prevents us from sleeping well at night, so we need it again to wake up—and so on. It therefore is recommended to decrease or avoid caffeine if you have sleep problems.

That said, some recent studies suggest that caffeine may be good for our brain. However, the long-term effects and optimal amounts are unknown at this time. Meanwhile numerous studies link coffee and tea consumption with better health. Because coffee and tea are derived from plants, they offer a rich source of phytonutrients—many of which are powerful antioxidants. Intriguing studies suggest that coffee and tea may decrease our risk of cancer, heart disease, diabetes, stroke, and dementia. Limited studies also propose that they may promote fat burning and lower cholesterol.

In particular green tea appears to help maintain good health. The benefits of green tea may be due to the fact that it is minimally processed. Unlike black and oolong teas, which are fermented, green tea leaves are withered and steamed, a process that retains high levels of phytonutrients. Compared to other teas and coffee, green tea is relatively low in caffeine. Most authorities say the average cup contains 15 to 40 milligrams of caffeine, while black tea has 40 to 80 milligrams, and coffee has over 100 milligrams per cup.

In short, the evidence suggests that enjoying tea and coffee can improve our health. It is unclear how many cups we should drink to reap these potential benefits. So it's best to decide based on how these beverages make you feel. Often we do not realize caffeine's negative effects until we actually cut back or eliminate it from our diet. For those who are sensitive to caffeine, green tea or decaffeinated teas and coffees are preferable. Although decaffeinated brews still contain some caffeine, the amount is relatively small, at 2 to 4 milligrams per cup. A natural decaffeination process is best for avoiding chemical residues, and though it may remove some of the phytonutrients, at least you won't be overstimulated.

Fizzle Out Soda

f I could pick one beverage that you should immediately remove from your diet, it would be soda. Its high sugar content will cause a spike in blood sugar and insulin, and the high fructose corn syrup that is a frequent ingredient promotes abdominal fat and increased lipids. Cola, one of the most popular soft drinks, is particularly damaging to our bones. The Framingham Osteoporosis study in 2006 concluded that women who drank cola had a decrease in their bone mineral density. It is believed that the phosphoric acid in cola leaches calcium from our bones and contributes to osteoporosis. Did you know that cola can be used to remove rust from metal and clean toilets? Think about what it does to your teeth. The phosphoric acid in cola eats away at tooth enamel and increases the risk of dental erosion. This is true even for diet colas. Do you need any more reasons to give it up? Your smile, your bones, and your brain will thank you when you phase out the fizzy drinks.

A NEW TWIST ON MARTINIS

Although much has been written about how red wine in moderation can be good for your heart and your brain, I would like you to reconsider. It's important to understand that the studies supporting this claim are "observational." This means they were conducted through self-reported questionnaires inquiring into the drinking habits of a large group of people, then correlated with their heart and brain health. Let's look at why these types of studies may be severely flawed and why the opposite conclusion—that moderate drinking is unhealthy—may, in fact, be true.

In recent years we have seen that the results of similar "observational" studies were disproved when subjected to a "randomized controlled trial"—the standard bearer of scientific proof. A good example of this is female hormone replacement. For decades it was believed that female hormone replacement was beneficial. But a randomized controlled trial, called the Women's Health Initiative, demonstrated that the exact opposite was true. The study was stopped in 2002 because women taking the study pills of estrogen plus progestin were developing heart disease and breast cancer at increased rates compared to those taking the placebo or inactive pills.

Unfortunately, randomized control trials have not been done on alcohol, nor are they likely to be done in the near future. And there is reason to believe that the observational studies out there are flawed. An important study by Dr. Tim Naimi looked at the characteristics between moderate drinkers and teetotalers. He found that moderate drinkers were wealthier, healthier, better educated, and received better health care than those who abstained from alcohol. In other words, there are many other reasons why moderate drinkers are healthier that may have nothing to do with alcohol.

Additionally, in his editorial for the *New England Journal of Medicine*, Dr. Ira Goldberg wrote: "One wonders if the alcohol consuming group also drank more tea, ate more nuts or consumed more fish." So we would be wise to think twice before toasting to the health of our brains with alcohol.

There have also been news stories about the incredible antioxidant benefits of resveratrol, which is found in red wine. This has been used by spirits' fans and distributors as yet another reason to fill our goblets. Although studies did show mice that were given hefty doses of resveratrol were healthier and lived longer, an article in the *New York*

Times pointed out that the average 150-pound person would need to drink 750 to 1,500 bottles of red wine a *day* in order to get the equivalent beneficial dose!

One thing that is not in dispute, however, is the fact that alcohol is a neurotoxin. Excess alcohol causes widespread damage throughout the nervous system, and in particular, it kills off cells in important memory areas. When intake is not curbed, alcoholic dementia ensues. A 2004 study by Changhai Ding and colleagues using MRI imaging showed that moderate alcohol intake is associated with brain atrophy. Even more brain damage may occur in teenagers who binge drink, because their brains are not yet fully developed.

It is also important for women to take into account the fact that even low to moderate alcohol consumption is associated with an increased risk of cancer. Although previous studies have shown a link between alcohol consumption and breast cancer, the Million Women Study in the UK shows that women who drink as little as one alcoholic beverage per day, be it wine, beer, or hard liquor, have an increased risk of cancer. The risk increased with increasing alcohol consumption, especially for cancers of the breast, liver, mouth, throat, and esophagus. After reviewing this study for the *Journal of the National Cancer Institute*, Michael Lauer, M.D., and Paul Sorlie, Ph.D., of the National Heart, Lung and Blood Institute in Bethesda, Maryland, concluded: "From a standpoint of cancer risk, the message of this report could not be clearer. There is no level of alcohol consumption that can be considered safe."

Although the above study is also observational, taking all this information into account, as well as the dire consequences of alcohol abuse and addiction, as far as I'm concerned the conclusion is clear: Alcohol is not good for us, even in small amounts. So if you can't give up that glass of wine with dinner, a Smart Diet would include reducing the amount of alcohol you drink. If you need even more incentive for a last call, remember that alcohol contains empty calories that slow the body's ability to burn fat for energy, and some studies support the notion that binge drinking can promote abdominal fat. They don't call it a beer belly for nothing!

Food-Triggered Headaches

If you suffer from headaches or migraines, you might want to pay attention to what you're eating and drinking. Both dietary habits and specific foods can trigger headaches. Keeping a food and beverage diary can be helpful in pinpointing the cause. Some common dietary habits that cause headache are dehydration, fasting, and skipping meals. Others include drinking alcohol, especially red wine; aged cheese (for example, Swiss, Parmesan, and cheddar); food additives such as MSG and nitrites; chocolate; and artificial sweeteners. We can't look or feel our best when we have headaches, so do whatever you can to find out what's causing them.

THE TRUTH ABOUT SUPPLEMENTS

It seems every month there's some new nutritional miracle making headlines, such as the antioxidant alpha lipoic acid, which claims to destroy free radicals in your cells, or acai berry, a Brazilian fruit that is professed to help with weight loss, sleep problems, and even sexual dysfunction. Some even claim that certain nutrients can cure cancer and other diseases. The problem is these claims have no scientifically controlled studies that back them up.

The myth about supplements is that they pick up the nutritional slack when our daily dietary needs are not met, and that they contain some herb or substance that will make us stronger and healthier. Herbal remedies and supplements have become a $25-billion-a-year industry, and as much as we would like a magic elixir that will enhance our memory and add years to our lives, study after study shows that most dietary supplements don't work.

Even more disturbing is a recent report finding that nearly all of the herbal dietary supplements tested in a congressional investigation contained trace amounts of lead and other contaminants. Although the levels of heavy metals, including mercury, cadmium, and arsenic, did not exceed thresholds considered dangerous, sixteen of the forty supplements tested contained pesticide residues that appeared to exceed legal limits. In some cases the government has not set allowable levels of these pesticides, because of a lack of scientific research.

At least nine products that made seemingly illegal health claims included a product containing ginkgo biloba that was labeled as a treatment for Alzheimer's disease. While ginkgo biloba, ginseng, and other supplements are touted to enhance memory and benefit dementia, none of these claims are supported by good clinical studies. Believe me, if they were proven to be beneficial, all neurologists and physicians who care for patients with Alzheimer's disease would be prescribing them.

Taking care of patients helps me stay on my toes about the latest supplement trends. They ask me about coenzyme Q10, ginseng, beta-carotene, resveratrol, selenium, lutein, ginkgo biloba, alpha lypoic acid, polyphenols, phosphatidylserine, DMAE—to name just a few popular supplements on the market. My advice is simple: Eat a rich variety of fruits and vegetables instead. While good scientific studies on supplements are limited, numerous studies show that eating a healthful diet does have a powerful impact on your health and can reduce your risk of memory loss and Alzheimer's disease. The truth is, by following the Smart Diet you should be getting all the nutrients that your body and your brain needs. Not only is it safer, but it's also a whole lot cheaper!

Here are some things to consider when it comes to supplements.

✦ Supplements are not regulated and monitored by the FDA like prescription or over-the-counter drugs, so many of the manufacturer's claims about safety and efficacy are unproven. There are thousands of supplements on the market, and very few have been well studied. As a result they may have some hidden or unknown side effects.

✦ Although many dietary supplements are from plant sources, "natural" does not always mean safe. The herbs comfrey and kava, for example, can cause serious harm to the liver. Beware of the marketing hype that splashes "natural" on just about anything to fool the consumer into believing it's healthy.

✦ Because there is no regulation, supplements may contain dozens of unknown compounds and active ingredients. In other words, what's on the label might not be what's in the bottle, so the amount of the active ingredient might be lower or higher than stated. As we mentioned above, a dietary supplement can be contaminated with other herbs, lead, pesticides, or metals, or even adulterated with unlabeled ingredients such as prescription drugs.

✦ Supplements can interact with one another and with prescription drugs. Because they are not closely monitored or studied, we may not be aware of these interactions. For example,

Saint-John's-wort, an herbal remedy taken for depression, can have serious side effects if taken with prescription antidepressant medications.

However, there are some tried and true vitamins and supplements that have been proven to be both safe and effective that I do recommend for some patients. I suggest buying them from a reputable manufacturer, especially one that your doctor or pharmacist recommends. As we said in Step three, Mind Your Body, always consult your healthcare provider before taking any supplements.

✦ **Fish oil.** If you don't like, or can't eat, oily fish twice a week, you might want to try fish oil. But make sure to talk to your doctor first. Emerging research suggests fish oil supplements may have a place in the prevention and treatment of Alzheimer's, depression, and other brain disorders. The evidence is strongest for heart disease. The American Heart Association recommends 1 gram daily of fish oils, but only for those with heart disease, and higher doses for those with high triglycerides. Good studies also support the use of 1 gram daily of fish oil for arthritis.

✦ **Vitamin D.** There has been a tremendous amount of research on vitamin D and the brain in the last few years. Low levels have been linked to poor cognitive function, dementia, stroke, depression, and multiple sclerosis. In addition to its traditional role in bone health, emerging evidence also suggests it's important for cardiovascular health and cancer prevention.

You can get vitamin D by eating oily fish like salmon, mackerel, bluefish, catfish, sardines, and tuna, as well as cod liver and fish oils. Dairy products are another great source of vitamin D. Sometimes called the sunshine vitamin, ten to fifteen minutes of unprotected sunlight exposure daily naturally boosts levels. If you are eating a Smart Diet and spending time outdoors (which is part of your brain makeover program), you are probably getting enough of your required dose.

There are many factors that increase our risk of vitamin D deficiency, including living in northern regions where there is less sunlight, having dark skin, certain antiseizure medications, advanced age, renal disease, and lactase deficiency. Most physicians recommend calcium with vitamin D supplements for postmenopausal women to prevent osteoporosis. I strongly recommend that you discuss this with your personal physician. Vitamin D deficiency can be easily diagnosed by a simple blood test.

+ **B12.** B12 deficiency is a recognized cause of poor cognitive function or one of the so-called reversible causes of dementia. People with poor memory or cognitive decline should have their B12 level checked. Some people are unable to absorb this important vitamin despite a high dietary intake or taking a B12 supplement. In these cases, a B12 injection is required. B12 deficiency can be readily diagnosed by a serum blood test.

+ **Multivitamins and folate.** For women in their reproductive years who may become pregnant, it is essential to have adequate amounts of folate and other vitamins for healthy fetal development. Folate deficiency during pregnancy is associated with serious fetal brain and nervous system defects. Prenatal vitamins are recommended for all women planning to become pregnant and should be continued throughout pregnancy. Women past their childbearing years who consume a healthy diet do not need to take a multivitamin, though many choose to do so for added assurance.

YOUR SMART DIET TAKE-AWAY

Once you are in the right mind-set and are following the Smart Diet, you will see your brain and body undergo an amazing transformation. The Smart Diet guidelines will provide your brain with all the nutrients and building blocks it needs to keep it functioning at its best. Some key points to remember:

- ✦ Make colorful vegetables, legumes, fruits, and whole grains the mainstay of every meal.

- ✦ Have fatty fish at least twice a week, and enjoy other safe fish and seafood regularly.

- ✦ Prepare foods with monounsaturated oils (olive, peanut, sesame, and canola).

- ✦ Use a rich variety of spices and herbs instead of salt.

- ✦ Enjoy multiple small servings of low-fat dairy every day.

- ✦ Limit poultry and eggs to twice a week.

- ✦ Save meats and sweets for special occasions.

- ✦ Drink water, teas, and coffee. No soda!

- ✦ Use alcohol sparingly, though none may be best.

GET READY TO BEAUTIFY
YOUR BRAIN RHYTHMS

In the final step, we will explain why getting enough "beauty sleep" will not only improve your memory and mood but also renew and regenerate your cells from head to toe. This final step of your beauty/ brain makeover will focus on tuning in to your natural circadian rhythms—the secret to rejuvenating sleep. You will learn how deep, restorative sleep will regulate your hormonal levels, restore your brain's energy, and make you feel refreshed and ready to face a new day!

Beautify Your Brain Rhythms

Everything has rhythm. Everything dances.
—MAYA ANGELOU, POET

During this final step in our beauty/brain makeover, you will learn how regulating your brain rhythms will profoundly improve your mental clarity, health, well-being, and appearance. What do we mean by "brain rhythms"? Deep in our brain are two tiny clocks that orchestrate our daily "circadian rhythms"—the twenty-four-hour tempo and pulse that determines our sleep/wake cycles. In synchrony with these clocks, hormones are secreted at precise intervals, regulating cellular activity throughout our body. If you have ever experienced jet lag, you know what it feels like when your circadian rhythms are out of synch. Even minor disturbances in our brain rhythms can have rippling effects on our ability to function properly and make us more susceptible to disease.

It's no accident that we call it "beauty rest" or that we must "sleep on it" when making important decisions. Getting a good night's sleep not only helps to regulate our brain rhythms, but it also sharpens our memory, lifts our mood, and helps us look our best. Did you know, for example, that the eye movements that occur while we're dreaming actually improve the circulation around our eyes, which helps us get rid of those dark circles we get when we're sleep deprived? This is just one reason why sleeping, and especially dreaming, is such an important part of our beauty/brain makeover.

ARE YOU GETTING ENOUGH "BEAUTY REST"?

There is actual scientific evidence behind the old wives' tale that we need our "beauty rest" in order to look our best. The truth is, sleep can lessen the severity of wrinkles in our face and neck—at least temporarily. This is due in part to the decline in body temperature and the shift of fluid within our body as we sleep. Lying down diverts the force of gravity—and we all know what gravity does to our face over time! Before bedtime, our body cools approximately a half a degree; in order to do this, our circulatory system increases blood flow to the skin. This produces a flush in our cheeks at night (similar to the flush we get when we exercise). We also tend to perspire more during sleep, which acts as a natural moisturizer that smoothes out wrinkles.

It is when we are fast asleep that we get the most benefits from our beauty rest. This is because our beautifying growth hormone, which repairs and rebuilds body tissues, including skin, muscle, and bone, is primarily secreted during the deepest phase of sleep. In response to the growth hormone that is released from the pituitary (a small gland suspended from the brain), our skin cells begin to regenerate faster at night than during the day—peaking at around 2:00 A.M. Our cells also increase their production of proteins as we sleep. Because proteins are the building blocks necessary for cell growth and for the repair of damage that comes from stress and too much sun, deep sleep is truly one of the best rejuvenating skin treatments.

RIDING YOUR BRAIN WAVES

By placing a series of electrodes on the scalp, we can record the brain waves that show the electrical activity of our brain. This tool, called an electroencephalogram or "EEG," allows us to see the distinctive rhythms of the human brain. When we are awake and relaxed there will be repetitive waves, between eight and thirteen per second, called "alpha rhythms." As we fall asleep, alpha waves give way to new brain rhythms in a similarly predictable time pattern.

Through brain-wave analysis we have come to understand the different stages of sleep. Although it may seem as though our brain is quiet during deep slumber, it actually goes through a roller coaster cycle of activity. Each sleep cycle is composed of a dream stage called REM (rapid eye movement), and three stages without dreaming called non-REM. As drowsiness sets in, the alpha rhythm of wakefulness is replaced by slower "theta" waves. This is called stage 1 sleep. It is the lightest stage, from which we are easily aroused, and lasts only a few minutes.

Stage 2 follows, characterized by the appearance of "sleep spindles" and "K complexes" on the brain wave tracing. After five to fifteen minutes, brain rhythms transition to stage 3, sometimes called "deep sleep" or "slow wave sleep." Stage 3, the deepest period of sleep, has dramatically high peaks and low troughs. These high rolling waves slowly crest between one to four times per second. It is difficult to awaken someone during this stage, which can last up to thirty minutes.

We then drift back to the lighter stage 2 before REM sleep finally makes its first appearance with the fast rhythms and rapid eye movements for which it was named. This symphony of brain waves completes the first cycle of sleep. We typically go through four to six sleep cycles in the course of the night, with an average cycle lasting about ninety minutes. As the night progresses, we spend less time in the deep slow-wave sleep of stage 3, and as morning approaches we spend more time in REM sleep.

Remarkably, the brain wave activity during REM is nearly indistinguishable from that of a mind that is fully awake. In fact, during REM sleep the brain uses more energy than when it is awake and concentrating on a difficult problem. While we don't fully understand REM sleep and the purpose of dreaming, we do know that our brain craves it. If someone is deprived of REM sleep, they will experience "REM rebound" and spend more time in dream sleep in subsequent nights when sleep is undisturbed. Some scientists believe that creativity is fostered during REM sleep, and inspiration often comes after awakening. I know that some of my best ideas have come after a good night's rest!

TO SLEEP, PERCHANCE TO LEARN

Numerous studies have confirmed the crucial role sleep plays in memory consolidation and learning. We know, for instance, that sleep is vital for processing new information and for the long-term storage of memory. When my sons were young, I would tell them to get to bed early "so you'll remember everything you learned in school today!" As they got older and became eager to improve their athletic prowess, my new mantra was: "It's practice *with sleep* that makes perfect."

I was teaching them what I knew about the brain's ability to learn and hone new skills during sleep. Many studies have confirmed that our memory and our visual and motor skills improve after sleep. Studies by Harvard neuroscientists Drs. Matthew Walker and Robert Stickgold reveal that when motor skills are taught early in the morning and tested twelve hours later *before* bed, no improvement is noticed. But after a night of slumber, there was a 20 percent increase in speed and a 39 percent improvement in accuracy. And while most sleep-enhanced learning takes place the first night after training, subjects who had two consecutive nights of adequate sleep increased their speed by 26 percent and their accuracy to nearly 50 percent. Conversely, participants who had fewer than six hours of sleep after training showed no overnight improvement.

So how does the brain consolidate memory and learning during sleep? Research suggests that the brain reviews the events of the day during sleep. Dr. Matthew Wilson of MIT studied the electrical brain activity of mice while they negotiated a maze. He discovered that the exact same pattern of brain activity occurred during sleep. The recordings were made from single cells deep in the animals' hippocampal memory centers. It appears that the rats were replaying the memory of running through the maze while they slept.

And while we don't know if the rats were actually dreaming about the maze, we do know that dreaming can help people learn new skills. Scientists at Beth Israel Deaconess Medical Center in Boston trained approximately a hundred volunteers to wend their way on a virtual maze as quickly as possible. Then half the volunteers were allowed to sleep for ninety minutes, while the other half stayed awake reading or relaxing. After ninety minutes, the sleeping subjects were awakened and asked to describe their dreams. All participants were then asked to try the maze again. Those who hadn't napped showed no improvement or did worse after the break, while those who got shut-eye and didn't have any maze dreams did only marginally better. Notably, however, those nappers who reported having dreamed about the maze showed a marked improvement, cutting their completion time in half.

Brain imaging techniques such as functional MRI (fMRI) have also shown that the brain literally changes overnight. Comparing the brain activation pattern for a newly acquired motor skill both before and after sleep suggests that there is reorganization of neural networks during sleep. This supports the idea that learning is reinforced and strengthened while we slumber and that dreaming about a task or problem will help us solve it.

Power Naps

Naps are a great way to recharge our batteries and boost learning retention during the day, especially with longer naps, where we fall into a deep sleep. The best time for a nap tends to be after lunch, when we're more likely to feel a little drowsy due to a natural dip in our circadian rhythm. But this varies with different people, and some find getting forty winks during the day makes it more difficult to fall asleep at night. So, like most things, we need to listen to our bodies to decide what is best for us.

HORMONAL RHYTHM AND BLUES

Whether it's Mommy Brain, PMS, or Senior Moments, when our hormonal rhythm and sleep cycles are out of whack, we (and sometimes those around us) can suffer from the blues. Here are some stories that might sound familiar:

✦ Mariko, a new mother, gets up every three hours during the night to breast-feed her son. The baby starts crying again at 5:00 A.M., and she can barely drag herself out of bed to tend to his needs. She feels as though her mind, which was once rapier sharp, has morphed into a mushier version of its former self. Her Mommy Brain caused her to forget to pack her older child's lunch and to snap at her husband for not making breakfast as he had promised. She looks at herself as she passes a mirror and realizes that she hasn't washed her hair in days. She glances droopy-eyed at the living room, where she is too exhausted to pick up the toys strewn all over the floor. Inside her throbbing head she worries: "What has happened to my life!? Will I ever be my old self again?"

✦ Cassandra, thirty, is always in motion—running, biking, working out—and working long hours as a fund-raiser for a non-profit organization. The only thing that stops Cassandra in her tracks is PMS. Like clockwork, the week before her period begins she'll start feeling cranky, crampy, and bloated. Her PMS is so bad that all she can do is curl up with a blanket in front of the TV with a heating pad. Her boyfriend has even marked these PMS days on his calendar so he knows to steer clear of her until her emotional storm passes.

✦ Zuri started getting hot flashes after she turned fifty-three. After not having her period for more than a year, suddenly her face would flush beet red as sweat trickled down her neck. If she is home during one of her flashes, she'll stick her head in the freezer, using a package of frozen peas as a pillow until the heat dies down. At night Zuri awakes to find her cotton top drenched like some middle-aged wet T-shirt contest. After changing shirts she manages to drift back to sleep only to be awakened again by the feeling that her body is on fire. The next day she is tired and irritable. She can't remember the last time she had any desire to be intimate with her husband.

✦ Betty is a healthy, active seventy-nine-year-old widow. She enjoys playing with her grandkids and going out to lunch with her fellow retired teachers once a week. As much as she likes this time in her life, she finds it impossible to get more than five hours of sleep a night. Betty will try to lull herself to sleep by listening to the radio or by taking sleep aids, but inevitably she will get up several times to go to the bathroom and find it difficult to fall back to sleep. Her lack of rest makes it necessary to nap during the day, and Betty also finds that she can no longer recall names and phone numbers of old friends that once rolled easily off her tongue. She calls these lapses her Senior Moments.

Whatever our age or stage of life, hormonal cycles and brain rhythms affect our moods, memory, and biologic functions. Like the sleep/wake cycle, hormones are secreted in rhythmic pulses in synch with our twenty-four-hour circadian rhythm. The so-called sleep hormone, melatonin, has circulating levels that vary during this daily cycle. It rises in the evening, making us sleepy, and peaks in the early morning, hours before we awaken. Melatonin secretion is regulated by light exposure. Our brain produces melatonin primarily at night, and levels drop in the presence of daylight. However, it's important to know that artificial light, especially the blue part of the spectrum that emanates from computer screens, TVs, and fluorescent bulbs, can also suppress melatonin secretion. In addition to being a powerful antioxidant, known for its antiaging benefits, melatonin also appears to play an important role in synaptic plasticity and memory.

Meanwhile other hormones regulate a variety of functions, including leptin and ghrelin (appetite); insulin (energy storage), and thyroid hormones (metabolism), all of which follow a unique circadian pattern of secretion. For example, growth hormone, which is essential for growth and cellular regeneration, is rhythmically secreted at night during stage 3 slow wave sleep. Similarly, our female hormones, including estrogen, progesterone, FSH, and LH, oscillate over a twenty-four-hour period. The dance of female hormones varies from menarche, when menstruation begins, to menopause, and changes yet again when we are pregnant or lactating. The complex interplay of the rhythmic cycling of all these hormones (and many more that I didn't even mention!) is exquisitely timed by our brain's biological clocks.

If you want to fully achieve a brain makeover you must maintain the right hormonal balance through regular sleep/wake cycles. As with Mariko, Cassandra, Zuri, and Betty, the toll that sleep loss takes on our health when our circadian rhythms and hormonal levels are out of synch can make us confused, irritable, and prone to feeling anxious and depressed.

The Sleepy Brain Drain

As I mentioned earlier, when the brain is sleep deprived, all domains of cognitive function are impaired, including concentration, memory, and judgment. Lack of sleep will slow down our reflexes and the speed that we process information, which causes us to make mistakes and increases our risk of having accidents. A sobering study by Dr. Drew Dawson compared the cognitive impairment effects of sleep deprivation to the effects of alcohol consumption. They found that after seventeen hours of sustained wakefulness, performance impairment was equivalent to that of a blood alcohol concentration of 0.05 percent. After twenty-four hours of wakefulness, it was equivalent to a blood alcohol level of 0.1 percent. Given that the blood alcohol level for legal intoxication is 0.08 percent, driving when sleepy is *as* dangerous as driving under the influence.

BEAUTY SLEEP

Sleep deprivation is not only bad for our brain, but it can also age us and make us fat. Chronic sleep deprivation and irregular sleep/wake cycles result in dark eye circles, dull skin, and weight gain. This is because the beautifying hormonal surges and bodily repair treatments that are scheduled to take place during sleep have to be put on hold. Missing out on sleep is like canceling an expenses-free trip to the best spa in town. But the effects of sleep deprivation are much more than just skin deep.

Sleep deprivation also sets the stage for countless medical problems, including high blood pressure, heart disease, diabetes, unhealthy cholesterol and triglyceride levels, a weakened immune system, and an increased risk for infections. As you know from Step three, many of these conditions lead to poor cognitive function and even dementia.

In fact, recent research suggests that sleep deprivation may be linked to Alzheimer's disease. In one study, chronic sleep deprivation increased amyloid beta plaque formation in mice—one of the hallmarks of Alzheimer's disease. Although the underpinnings of this relationship are still unknown, the take-home message is clear: Regular sleep/wake cycles are essential for keeping your brain healthy and functioning at its best.

How do our brain clocks work? On the undersurface of your brain behind the bridge of your nose, two small clusters of neurons called the suprachiasmatic nuclei (SCN) generate your twenty-four-hour circadian rhythm. This master rhythm maker regulates our sleep/wake cycle and hormonal rhythms, and sets the pulse and pace of cellular activity. Special light receptors in the retina feed directly into the SCN, keeping our clocks in tune with the outside world. These pathways are particularly sensitive to natural light, though artificial light also affects them. There is increasing concern about how artificial light at night disrupts our natural circadian rhythms and its potential link to breast cancer.

Scientists have known for years that rats raised in cages where the lights are left on all night are 60 percent more likely to get breast cancer than when the light is turned off. There is mounting evidence that this might also be true in humans. Women who do shift work (for example, nurses, factory workers, and flight attendants) report more frequent menstrual disturbances and have an increased risk of breast cancer.

Equally alarming is a study that used satellite images of Earth and cancer registries to discover that women who live in neighborhoods with large amounts of nighttime illumination also appear to have increased rates of breast cancer. It is also well known that women who are completely blind and are unable to perceive light have a lower risk of contracting breast cancer than sighted women.

How do we put this all together? Scientists believe that artificial light at night disrupts our SCN even when we're sleeping. You see, the SCN is exquisitely sensitive to light. So whether we're awake doing shift work or asleep with our eyes closed, artificial light at night upsets our brain clocks. And as you now know, when our SCN is out of synch, all our hormonal pulses are out of step, including melatonin and female hormones. Melatonin is thought to have tumor-inhibiting properties. The combined disruption of normal melatonin and female hormonal secretion is believed to trigger breast cancer.

This mounting concern prompted the World Health Organization to classify shift work as a "probable carcinogen" on a par with toxic chemicals such as PCBs. Given what we now know, women should be even more vigilant about maintaining regular sleep/wake cycles and limiting exposure to artificial light at night. If you are unable to darken your sleeping area, a sleep mask is the perfect solution.

Light Up Your Mind

Nature is intrinsically timed to the alternating rhythm of light and dark produced by Earth's rotation. Cicadas chirp, birds sing, and blossoms open and close in tune with this twenty-four-hour cycle. Daylight also paces the activity of our mind. When deprived of regular intervals of dark and light, the mind can lose its bearings. This is especially true with elderly people for whom brain function is already compromised. For example, some older people who function fine at home can become confused when hospitalized where artificial lighting is on 24/7. While there are often other contributing factors, such as underlying illness and medications, the loss of rhythmic light and dark exposure will only worsen their condition. Simply moving the patient to a bed that is near a window and darkening the room at night can significantly improve mental clarity.

BRIGHTEN YOUR BRAIN

Shakespeare said it well when he wrote about "the winter of our discontent." He didn't know it at the time, but there is biological reason why our moods are sunnier during the spring and summer. Seasonal affective disorder (SAD) is a form of depression that sets in during the winter months when sunlight wanes. Like other forms of depression, SAD occurs more commonly in women and should be treated by a mental health professional. Most women who develop the "winter blahs" or "cabin fever" do not have SAD, but getting more sunlight will help us all feel better. Here's what you can do during the dark winter months:

+ Spend more time outside during daylight. Don't forget the sunscreen if you're out for longer than ten minutes— too much sun can cause premature wrinkles and make you vulnerable to skin cancers.

+ Arrange your home and office furniture to spend more time in sunny areas when working.

+ Strategically add mirrors to your living space to reflect light and brighten up your surroundings.

+ Keep your curtains and blinds open during the day.

+ Consider investing in a light therapy box. (See the sidebar on the next page.)

Light Therapy Boxes

Although there's nothing like the real thing, light therapy boxes emit bright light that simulates sunshine. You can buy a light therapy box over the counter, but do your homework first. There are many types and styles available and not all of them have been tested for safety and efficiency. Avoid those that do not filter out harmful UV light. Never look directly at the light source, and be sure to get one that can be positioned appropriately above your line of vision. Choose one that is specifically designed for SAD to ensure that the light will be in the correct range. Light intensity also varies. Some boxes give off only the preferred intensity of 10,000 lux within a few inches of the source, while others extend beyond two feet. If you plan to use one in different places, you should get one that is portable. Some come with programmable timers that simulate dawn—turning on in the morning while you're asleep and becoming brighter as you wake up.

SLEEPLESS NIGHTS

There are two general types of insomnia: transient and chronic. Approximately forty million Americans suffer from chronic insomnia each year, according to the Association for Neurological Disorders and Stroke, and an additional twenty million experience occasional sleeping problems. Transient insomnia is typically brought on by short-term stress, anxiety, excitement over an upcoming event, deadlines, temporary financial problems, or family concerns. Jet lag, work schedule shifts, and late nights out can also cause transient insomnia by disrupting our circadian rhythm. This kind of sleeplessness is short-lived, lasting only a few days or weeks, and does not have long-term consequences.

Insomnia is considered chronic when it lasts for months or years. It often waxes and wanes in severity and becomes more pronounced with situational stressors. There are many causes of chronic insomnia and often multiple contributing factors. If you can't remember the last time you got a good night's sleep, get evaluated by a doctor to determine the underlying cause. The reason you can't get shut-eye could be behavioral, environmental, emotional, or medical. Whatever the cause, it's a serious problem that you should not ignore.

How Much Sleep Is Enough?

While most experts say eight hours of sleep is ideal, the truth is it all depends on how you feel. Some people do well with seven hours or less, while others require nine or more to be at their best. If you are ill or under tremendous stress, you will probably need to sleep longer than you usually do. A woman's sleep needs also may vary, depending on her age, menstrual cycle, pregnancy, and menopause. Although the amount of sleep we get is important, the *quality* of our slumber is just as important.

The best indicator of how much sleep you need should be based on how you feel and how well you function. Keep in mind that sometimes we fool ourselves into thinking that we're getting enough sleep. If you are getting sufficient sleep, you should feel refreshed and not have trouble getting out of bed in the morning. You should also feel naturally alert throughout the day without the help of a caffeine boost.

RESET YOUR BRAIN CLOCKS

There are various ways to fight insomnia, starting with establishing a regular circadian rhythm. And one of the best ways to do this is by regulating your light exposure. As an experiment, close your eyes for a moment. Is everything pitch-black, or does a bit of light still come through? As you see, even with our eyes closed our brain can sense low levels of light. Brain clocks don't run on a perfect twenty-four-hour cycle and, like all timepieces, need to be reset every now and then. By knowing when to increase or decrease your light exposure, you can keep your brain clocks running on time as well as harmonize your hormones. The main idea is to get more bright light in the morning and avoid it in the evening.

How to Suppress Melatonin during the Day

◆ **Let the sun shine in.** Into your brain, that is. First thing in the morning, open the curtains and pull up the shades. If possible, go outside. This simple act will suppress melatonin secretion throughout the day. Doing this every morning at the same time is the best way to get your brain clock in synch.

✦ **Light up your face.** If you live in a dark region of the country or wake up before sunrise, use a makeup mirror when getting ready in the morning. Find one that simulates daylight, or consider purchasing a light therapy box (see page 218).

✦ **Lose the shades.** In the morning, whether you are out with your dog, commuting to work, or just walking to your car, don't wear sunglasses, for another added boost of melatonin suppression. (Keep them on at midday when the sun is bright, however, to protect your eyes.) Short spurts of unprotected sunlight will do the trick.

How to Boost Melatonin at Night

✦ **Wind down.** Get in the habit of preparing your brain for sleep by winding down activity in the evening and going to bed at the same time every night.

✦ **Shut off the TV and computer.** Save your e-mailing for the morning and record your favorite late-night talk shows and watch them earlier in the evening if you want to get to sleep. The high-frequency blue light emitted from these screens will keep you up by keeping your melatonin down.

✦ **Change your lightbulbs.** Avoid bright and fluorescent lights before bedtime. For those lamps you use in the evening, replace bright lightbulbs with incandescent low-wattage bulbs, which are less stimulating.

✦ **Cover your electrical displays.** Our bedrooms are often lit up with tiny lights coming from our alarm clocks, DVDs, telephones, and other electrical gadgets. Cover them up before you go to bed to keep the room dark. (If you must have some light in the room, low-frequency red lights are preferable.)

✦ **Use a flashlight.** Don't switch on the light if you go to the bathroom at night. Use a flashlight instead, or get a light dimmer so it's easier to get back to sleep. Please do not do this if you are unsteady on your feet!

✦ **Keep the bedroom dark.** Use heavy curtains or shades to block out incoming light, or consider wearing a sleep mask. The darker the room, the deeper you will sleep.

STAYING IN SYNCH

While light exposure is the most important factor in keeping your circadian rhythms in snych, other steps in your brain makeover also play a role.

✦ **Physical activity.** Our circadian rhythms are designed for daytime activity and nighttime sleep, so regular physical activity will help keep your brain clocks running on time. A study on simulated jet lag showed that daily exercise accelerated the resetting of the sleep/wake cycle compared to a control group that did not exercise. In addition, physical activity tires out the body and reduces stress, both of which help promote drowsiness. Some experts advise morning workouts to boost our metabolism throughout the day, while others suggest the late afternoon, when our circadian body temperature peaks, making our muscles more supple and decreasing the risk of injury.

The short answer is it's really up to you. Some women prefer to exercise in the morning, while others find an evening workout the perfect segue into deep slumber. Be aware, however, that exercising too close to bedtime may make it difficult to fall asleep. Whatever works best for your lifestyle and whenever you feel most inclined to move should determine your exercise time.

✦ **Eating three squares.** Eating regular meals in tune with your circadian rhythms will help trim your waistline and harmonize your body chemistry. Our circadian rhythm synchronizes the metabolic processes throughout the body, including those involved in the burning and storage of energy. Remember insulin, the hormone that lowers blood sugar, from Step six? It is more effective at doing its job of lowering blood sugar in the morning than it is in the evening.

Therefore, if we're up snacking late at night, this means higher blood sugar and insulin spikes than we would have during the day. This leads not only to unhealthy inflammation but also to those extra calories being more likely to go to your waistline, as insulin promotes abdominal fat storage. On top of that, when food intake is out of synch with leptin and ghrelin, the hormones that regulate hunger and satiety, we're less likely to feel full, and we end up eating more. And then, when we do go to bed, we're not apt to sleep soundly because our tummies are so full. As you can see, this becomes a vicious cycle! So for a trim waistline and the sweetest slumbers, it is best to eat regular meals and avoid eating three hours before bedtime.

Sweet Dreams for Moms

When I resumed my medical training after maternity leave, I knew I would not be successful if my son wasn't sleeping well during the night. Fortunately, I read *Solve Your Child's Sleep Problems* by Dr. Richard Ferber, the director of Pediatric Sleep Disorders at Children's Hospital Boston. This landmark book is a *must* read for every mom. From dealing with difficulties falling asleep, to middle-of-the-night awakenings and night fears, this book provides safe and sound strategies to help your child fall asleep and stay asleep.

SLEEP BUSTERS

Remember the rhythmic ninety-minute sleep cycles that I described at the beginning of this step? When we monitor an individual's brain waves overnight (as is done in sleep labs), we get an elaborate tracing of brain wave activity. The overall picture of the sleep cycles, the stages of sleep contained within those cycles, along with the time spent in each stage, are called "sleep architecture." Many things can affect sleep integrity, causing our sleep architecture to become fragmented. When this happens, we miss out on the beautiful, rhythmic cycling of restorative sleep and feel miserable in the morning. The following are some common sleep busters:

✦ **Caffeine.** Caffeine from coffee, tea, and soft drinks can wreak havoc on your sleep/wake cycle and your sleep architecture. This is true even in small amounts and even if you only drink it in the morning! The reason for this is caffeine has a half-life of up to seven hours (the half-life is the time it takes for half of it to be metabolized). If you metabolize caffeine slowly and drink a cup of coffee in the morning, half of the caffeine will remain in your system seven hours later. And in another seven hours, when you're trying to fall asleep, one-quarter of the caffeine is still circulating in your system. The following morning one-eighth of the caffeine from the previous morning's cup of coffee is still in your system!

In addition, there are many factors that slow caffeine metabolism. As we get older, the effects of caffeine can linger even longer. Estrogen also slows caffeine clearance, meaning that a woman's sensitivity to caffeine may vary during her menstrual cycle. Similarly, the birth control pill, hormone replacement therapy, and other prescription medications can delay its metabolism, resulting in higher levels over longer periods of time. And as we previously mentioned, caffeine triggers the release of cortisol, the stress hormone, further interfering with our bodies' circadian rhythm. Therefore I always recommend that any women suffering from insomnia should decrease or abstain from caffeine. Don't forget that caffeine comes in many forms, including soda and chocolate, and is even in some over-the-counter medications.

✦ **Alcohol.** Many people have a nightcap, thinking it will help them sleep, but actually the opposite is true. Alcohol disrupts our sleep architecture, which becomes even more fragmented with excessive use. Alcoholics lack deep slow wave sleep, spend decreased time in REM sleep, and have frequent nighttime arousals. Even after years of abstinence, sleep disturbances can persist. Alcohol can have long-lasting effects on the brain, and for these reasons it should never be used as sleep aid.

✦ **Medications.** Take a look in your medicine cabinet if you are having trouble falling asleep, because your meds may be keeping you awake. The following are common medications that can cause insomnia and alter sleep architecture: antidepressants (buproprion, fluoxetine, venlafaxine); blood pressure meds (atenolol, propranolol, metoprolol); asthma meds (albuterol, theophylline); decongestants (pseudoephedrine, phenylpropanolamine); nicotine; steroids (prednisone); and stimulants (modafinil, methylphenidate, caffeine, dextroamphetamine). *Note*: Some over-the-counter and prescription analgesic medications contain caffeine, so check the ingredients.

Tucking In

Every mother knows that a nighttime routine will help ease a restless child into bed (for example, bath, book, bear hug, bed). The same applies to adults. Establish a regular bedtime routine, such as reading, writing (on paper!), or taking a warm bath by candlelight (try adding lavender, chamomile, sandalwood, or other essential oils known for their sleep-inducing scents). Do whatever it is you find relaxing.

Make sure your bedroom is conducive to sleep. It is easier to fall asleep in a cool room than in a hot one, so use an air conditioner during those sultry summer nights and keep the thermostat low in the wintertime. Wearing socks to bed can encourage your body temperature to drop, which will help you drift off to sleep. In addition to keeping the room dark, you might also want to wear earplugs to add to the sensory deprivation.

TREATING INSOMNIA

As we all know, one of the most common causes of insomnia is anxiety and stress. If you are concerned that you are not getting enough sleep, you might lie awake at night worrying about falling asleep, creating a vicious cycle of sleeplessness. In frustration, many people turn to over-the-counter sleep aids or prescription drugs for help. Although these medications can be effective in the short term, most of them have side effects, such as daytime drowsiness or mental clouding, and can interfere with the quality of your slumber.

Like alcohol, they can negatively impact sleep architecture. Although total sleep time may be increased, the quality of that sleep may be poor. Plus habitual sleep aid users often develop a tolerance to these medications, meaning that over time they lose their effectiveness. There is limited data on the safety of these medications during pregnancy, so if you are pregnant or trying to conceive it's best to keep the lid on the pill bottle.

✦ **Prescription hypnotics.** A variety of prescription medications called "hypnotics" are used to treat insomnia, including: zolpidem (Ambien), eszopiclone (Lunesta), ramelteon (Rozerem), zaleplon (Sonata), triazolam (Halcion), temazepam (Razepam, Restoril, Temaz). Their primary use is for transient sleep disruption due to jet lag, temporary stress, and environmental changes that keep you up at night. They may also be used for chronic insomnia when cognitive behavioral therapy and other treatments fail.

Hypnotics are prescribed based on the type of insomnia. For example, short-acting formulations work best for those who have trouble falling asleep, while long-acting agents work best for those with early morning awakening and daytime anxiety. As I said above, hypnotics can alter sleep architecture and sleep quality, and they can cause both physical and psychological dependence.

✦ **Antidepressants and antipsychotic medications.** Many of these medications have the side effect of sedation, but they should not be used primarily for treatment of insomnia as there is limited data regarding their efficacy for this condition. Examples include: trazodone, amitriptyline (Elavil), nortriptyline (Pamelor), quetiapine (Seroquel), risperidone (Risperdal) and mirtazapine (Remeron). Many of these medications alter sleep architecture and cause daytime drowsiness.

✦ **Diphenhydramine.** This is the most common over-the-counter sleep aid and is found in Tylenol PM and other formulations billed as sleep promoting. Also known by the brand name Benadryl, diphenhydramine is an antihistamine that commonly causes drowsiness. Its side effects include daytime sedation, dry mouth, and constipation. Because of its relatively long half-life, levels can build up if taken regularly and cause confusion. This is especially true in the elderly.

✦ **Melatonin.** Another over-the-counter agent, melatonin is commonly used for insomnia, particularly jet lag. As wonderful as our naturally produced melatonin is, the supplements are not monitored by the FDA, and data on long-term use is not yet available. There is, however, a new prescription medication called Rozerem (ramelteon) that works like melatonin by activating melatonin receptors. Unlike other sleep medicines, it is not thought to be habit forming. However, as with all medications, it should only be taken under a doctor's supervision.

✦ **Hormone replacement therapy.** Insomnia and excessive daytime sleepiness during perimenopause and menopause are most often caused by hot flashes and night sweats. In some circumstances, short-term use of hormone replacement therapy (HRT) can help alleviate these symptoms and improve sleep quality. There has been much discussion in the media about synthetic forms of hormones versus so called bio-identical hormones, but many women don't entirely understand the difference. Bio-identical hormones means you're getting the same exact hormones (estradiol and progesterone) that your body makes rather than a synthetic hormone that is similar but not exact.

While it makes sense that hormones that are the same as the ones your body produces would be best, there are no good studies available at this time to know if bio-identical hormones are any safer than the synthetic hormones. That said, your doctor *can* prescribe bio-identical hormones that are FDA approved and monitored. It is not advisable to use other types of nonprescription hormone therapy because, once again, you don't know what you're really taking. As always, the decision to use HRT should be made between you and your physician.

Reduce Wrinkles and Improve Your Posture While You Sleep

Did you know that the position in which you sleep can make you prone to wrinkles and poor posture? Sleeping on your back instead of on your stomach will help reduce wrinkles, according to the American Academy of Dermatologists. This makes sense when you think about it, because when you sleep on your stomach, your face is compressed between your pillow and the weight of your head, which creases the skin on your face. Similarly, sleeping on the same side every night can lead to wrinkles on that side of your face. So if you like to sleep on one particular side, be sure to switch sides each night.

Likewise, the position we sleep in can also adversely affect our posture. If you tend to round your shoulders and jut your head forward during the day, sleeping in a curled-up fetal position will only intensify this poor posture position. Similarly, sleeping on your stomach can exacerbate a swayback by allowing your lower back to sag into the mattress. The goal is to keep your spine and head aligned while you sleep.

For example, when sleeping on your side, it is important to have a firm pillow that will keep your head level with your spine and prevent your shoulder from rolling forward. If you must sleep on your stomach, placing a pillow under your abdomen will support your low back and prevent it from sagging into the mattress. Back sleepers can benefit from placing a small pillow under their knees, which flattens the lower back into a more neutral position, and a thin pillow under their head, so their face points toward the ceiling. They should also avoid sleeping on a stack of pillows, which will aggravate a slouching posture.

While sleeping on your back is optimal, be aware that it can aggravate sleep apnea (see page 234), which causes you to snore and disrupts your sleep. In the end, however, making adjustments to your sleeping position can improve your posture, skin appearance, and comfort during the night as well as during the day.

MAKE UP YOUR MIND TO SLEEP

By mastering the Relaxation Response (RR) and using the cognitive behavioral therapy (CBT) techniques we talked about in Step five, Make Over Your Mind, you can gain control over your mind, which will help you to overcome insomnia. Cognitive behavioral therapy has been clinically proven to be as effective as the hypnotic sleeping pills that I described above. Unlike medications, CBT does not lose its effectiveness over time. In fact, the more you practice, the more effective it will become. And the best part is—there are no side effects!

If you have trouble practicing this on your own, I strongly recommend that you try working with a licensed CBT therapist. Specify that your goal is to treat insomnia. It usually involves five to ten one-hour-long sessions to learn the essential skills to improve sleep that will be yours for a lifetime. Using the power of your own mind is the best way to enjoy beautifying brain waves all night long!

CONDITIONS THAT MAKE YOU TOSS AND TURN

If you are still unable to sleep despite trying CBT and efforts to synchronize your circadian rhythms, other causes need to be considered.

There are numerous physical ailments, medical conditions, and sleep disorders that can stop you from getting your much-needed slumber. Some are obvious and others may require an overnight sleep study in order for your doctor to make the diagnosis. During a sleep study, also called a "polysomnogram," brain waves, blood oxygen levels, muscle movements, and heart rate are monitored overnight in a sleep lab. Experts will review your study and relay the results to your doctor. I encourage you to work closely with your health professional to accurately diagnose your sleep problems. Your health and the quality of your life depend on it! The following are some common causes of sleep disruption and what you can do about them:

✦ **Pain.** There are many causes of pain at night, but nerve pain is one of the most common. Although we don't know why, nerve pain tends to become more severe at night. It most likely is due to changes in pain thresholds timed to our circadian rhythms. Peripheral neuropathy is the most common cause of nerve pain at night. It causes numbness, tingling, or a burning sensation in the hands and feet and is painful enough to keep even the most stoic among us from getting a restful sleep. People typically compare the loss of sensation to the feeling of wearing a thin stocking or glove. There are medications available that treat nerve pain that are not narcotics but work by dampening the firing of pain pathways. If this or any other kind of pain is interfering with your sleep, talk with your doctor to determine the underlying cause and best treatment. Please note that increased nocturnal bone pain can occasionally be a sign of cancer. Therefore always consult your physician for any unusual or unrelenting pain.

✦ **Frequent urination.** Getting up to use the bathroom numerous times during the night disrupts sleep continuity and quality.

For many women, this can simply be due to habit. If you empty your bladder frequently, it won't be used to holding urine at full capacity. Bladder training, a progressive program that teaches women to hold their urine for longer and longer periods during the day, can resolve this problem. For other causes of increased urination during the night, certain medications may be helpful and dramatically improve sleep quality. If frequent trips to the bathroom are disrupting your sleep, be sure to talk with your doctor.

✦ **Gastroesophageal reflux disease (GERD) or heartburn.** This common cause of insomnia, often referred to as GERD or acid reflux, is a condition in which stomach acid backs up or refluxes into the esophagus. The acid irritates the lining of the esophagus, causing discomfort and a burning sensation in the chest. Fortunately, there are measures you can take to improve symptoms. The first step is to avoid any aggravating factors such as smoking, alcohol use, and medications that irritate the stomach, including aspirin, ibuprofen, and naproxen. As always, consult with your doctor before stopping any prescribed medications. Eating dinner early in the evening, at least three to four hours before bedtime, or having smaller meals can be helpful, and avoiding spicy and acidic foods is also a good idea. To help prevent stomach acid from flowing upward during sleep, elevate the head of your bed by placing six- to eight-inch blocks under the bedposts. There are also many effective medications that you can take. As always, discuss with your doctor. Be aware that sometimes it is hard to tell the difference between acid reflux and chest pain originating from the heart. If there is any doubt, call 911.

✦ **Pregnancy.** The quality of our sleep tends to be most disrupted during the third trimester of pregnancy. Women may experience back pain, leg cramps, uncomfortable fetal movements, heartburn or acid reflux, pressure on the bladder, and, of course, the anxiety of impending childbirth! In some cases, obstructive sleep apnea may develop (see following). Physical therapy, stretching, and gentle exercise are helpful for back pain and leg cramps. You can also try invoking the Relaxation Response (repeating a word, phrase, or repetitive motion in a quiet place) to help ease your anxiety and cope with fetal movements and frequent urination. (For heartburn, see above.)

✦ **Obstructive sleep apnea.** In obstructive sleep apnea (OSA) the airway becomes intermittently blocked during sleep. When we're asleep, muscles throughout the body, including the throat, relax. In some cases, this can cause airway obstruction and the person stops breathing, which means blood oxygen levels fall. The low oxygen levels are sensed by the brain, which then rouses the individual. Often the sleeper will stir with a gasp and resume breathing without awakening. This can occur hundreds of times during the night, causing a marked fragmentation of sleep architecture. At times the person may awaken feeling panicked and short of breath. In the morning they feel tired and experience daytime sleepiness.

Many individuals with obstructive sleep apnea snore loudly. Being overweight increases the risk of developing OSA, and in women the risk increases during menopause. Various treatments are used, including aggressive weight loss, oral appliances that help keep the airway open, surgery to remove excess obstructive tissue around the airway, and continuous positive airway pressure (CPAP), which is a face mask that gently blows pressurized air into the airway to keep it open. If left untreated,

OSA causes *serious* health problems, including high blood pressure, heart failure, and memory loss. If you think that you or a loved one suffers from this condition be sure to seek medical advice and have a sleep study.

✦ **Perimenopause and menopause.** The hormonal fluctuations and declining estrogen and progesterone levels during perimenopause and menopause can cause a variety of symptoms that interfere with sleep/wake cycles. These include hot flashes, night sweats, insomnia, fatigue, and excessive daytime sleepiness. In addition to regulating circadian rhythms, women who exercise regularly and maintain a normal weight have fewer symptoms than those who are overweight and don't exercise. Avoid caffeine and alcohol, which disrupt your circadian rhythms and trigger hot flashes. Wearing moisture-wicking sleepwear and keeping the bedroom cool with a fan can be helpful. Some women find the Chillow—a pillow that stays cool at night—helps them sleep better. And in some cases, your doctor may prescribe hormone replacement therapy (see page 229) or other medications.

If the above measures don't work, something else might be causing your insomnia or excessive daytime fatigue. Obstructive sleep apnea in women dramatically increases with menopause. Menopause-associated weight gain could also be an underlying factor. As in Alison's case (see page 238), this can create a vicious cycle. When we are sleep deprived, we often lack the energy to exercise, which causes us to gain weight, which further exacerbates sleep apnea and other menopausal symptoms. So if you are having problems sleeping, be sure to see your doctor to get an accurate diagnosis and the proper treatment.

✦ **Restless legs syndrome.** If you have crawling sensations in your limbs at night associated with an irresistible urge to move your legs, you may have restless legs syndrome (RLS). This condition keeps people up walking the floors at night because only movement relieves these uncomfortable sensations. Consequently, people with this affliction suffer from significant sleep deprivation. RLS occurs in 1 percent to 5 percent of young to middle-aged adults, but increases to 10 percent to 20 percent of those over age sixty. Often there is no clear cause, and it tends to run in families. In some cases, however, underlying medical problems such as iron deficiency and renal failure can be the cause. Fortunately there are medications that effectively relieve the symptoms.

✦ **Periodic limb movement disorder.** In this sleep disorder, people are unaware that they have involuntary limb movements during sleep. These movements, which occur during non-REM sleep, cause the brain to arouse, even though they might not fully wake up. In the morning they still feel tired, as their sleep is not restorative, and they report excessive daytime sleepiness. Many go undiagnosed until a bed partner is awakened by the movements. Some medications can increase and even cause these symptoms, but effective treatments are available.

✦ **Advanced sleep phase syndrome (ASPS).** This condition is most common in older women. If you frequently awaken in the early morning, usually between 3:00 and 5:00 A.M., and have difficulty staying awake in the early evening, even in social settings, you might have ASPS. Fortunately this can be treated by using timed light exposure to reset your brain clock. Bright-light exposure in the early evening can suppress melatonin secretion, allowing you to stay awake later in the evening and eventually reset your circadian rhythm to a later hour.

✦ **Delayed sleep phase syndrome.** This is essentially the opposite of advanced sleep phase syndrome; the circadian pacemaker is set for a late bedtime with consequent awakening late in the morning. This pattern commonly occurs in teenagers and young adults, making it very hard to be attentive for early morning classes. Gradually advancing the awakening hour and treating the brain to bright-light exposure first thing in the morning usually does the trick.

✦ **Narcolepsy.** Rather than causing nighttime insomnia, this sleep disorder causes excessive daytime sleepiness. It is not unusual for people with narcolepsy to fall asleep in the midst of a conversation, while eating, or at the wheel. Unfortunately the latter is a common scenario. These "sleep attacks" or irresistible episodes of sleepiness occur suddenly and without warning. Symptoms usually start in adolescence or early adulthood. Narcolepsy is diagnosed by a special type of sleep study and treated with stimulants to keep the person alert during the day. While narcolepsy is not that common, there are many other causes of excessive daytime sleepiness. Being sleepy during the day is unhealthy and significantly increases the likelihood of accidents. If you or a loved one frequently nods off during the day, be sure to see a doctor.

Alison's Story

Alison, a business executive in her midfifties, came to see me for memory problems. She was having trouble focusing at work and was leaving out words in her memos and e-mails. Not only was she afraid that she was showing signs of early-onset Alzheimer's, but she was also concerned about losing her job when colleagues started noticing her errors. Although she was getting eight hours most nights, she felt tired upon awakening in the morning and often felt sleepy during the day. She attributed her fatigue to menopause and the twenty pounds she had put on over the past few years.

Because she lived alone, she didn't know if she snored, though she had on a few occasions awakened during the night gasping for air. I suspected that she had obstructive sleep apnea (OSA). Sleep apnea can be brought on when extra fat around the neck compresses the airway during sleep. An overnight sleep study confirmed my suspicions. Although Alison thought she was getting enough rest, the sleep apnea was preventing her from getting the deep, restorative sleep that she needed for optimal brain function. After using a continuous positive airway pressure machine (CPAP), which keeps airways open during the night, she saw a marked improvement in her memory and cognitive performance. Her energy level also improved, and she began exercising again, which she had given up due to the fatigue from sleep apnea. Over a year she was able to lose thirty pounds and no longer needed the CPAP. She was thrilled to be feeling "better than ever"!

SWEET DREAMS

Whatever is keeping you up at night, I hope this step has given you a better understanding of how important it is to harmonize your brain rhythms so you get enough of the restorative beauty rest you need to keep you feeling younger, smarter, and ready to face the new day!

By understanding more about how your brain works, and by heeding the advice in this book, I hope you will cherish and fully experience the joys of a beautiful, healthy brain. If you have followed the steps in this book, you should be sharper, healthier, and—yes—more beautiful! You have given yourself a new lease on life, and it shows in the way you look, act, and feel. And most important, you now possess the empowering skills to keep your brain beautiful for a lifetime.

I trust that you are enjoying your new brain and the new you. Is your mind clearer than it has been in years? Are people remarking that you appear happier, calmer, and prettier? Do you feel empowered by the new sense of control that you have over your mind and your life? Are you living more dynamically by indulging in heart-pumping, brain-enhancing movement and trying new things? Are you savoring your meals and taking time daily to read, relax, meditate, and engage in Passionate Pursuits?

I hope that you and your Beautiful Brain Buddies will spread the word to other women about the unlimited potential of their beautiful brain. I invite you to share the progress of your beauty/brain makeover by contacting me at www.mariepasinski.com. Please celebrate how far you've come and how much you have already learned. As you continue to follow this program, you will find that your Bad Brain Days will fade away and that many Beautiful Brain Days lie ahead!

ACKNOWLEDGMENTS

Countless beautiful minds have contributed to the writing of this book, and I thank you all for sharing your thoughts, experiences, and knowledge. To Karin Stanley, who first suggested this venture and has encouraged me every step of the way. You are a true artist whose creativity inspires those around you. To Anna (Betty) Brack, for sharing your life wisdom, which is always dispensed with a dose of humor. Special thanks to my supportive circle of remarkable women friends (aka The Goddesses): Ute Gfrerer, Rebecca Flacke, Mary Flannery, Suzanne Tarlov, Diane Dunfy, Cora Long, Christine Kendall, Patty Forster, and especially Louise Rusk for bringing us together, and my deepest gratitude to Linda Hall, who skillfully critiqued my drafts. Thank you, Linda, for always being there to brainstorm with an open door, a warm heart, and a cup of tea.

I am deeply indebted to all of my patients from whom I have learned so much and, more important, who have enriched my life and made it more meaningful. And to all the brilliant minds in medicine at Harvard and beyond who have so generously shared their knowledge and expertise over the years. Special thanks to Dr. Shahram Khoshbin for sharing your love of all things neurological and inspiring me to become a neurologist. Drs. David Dawson, Misha Pless, Tim Naimi, Seth Schonwald, Martin Samuels, Charles Barlow, Herbert Benson, Roger Sweet, Barbara Dworetzky, and Lorinda de Zayas also deserve an extra nod of thanks. To Sheila Arsenault and Deb Mahoney, two outstanding nurses whom I have been privileged to work

243

beside, thank you for nurturing my soul (and sense of humor) and for the wonderful care you give to our patients.

A special thanks to the women at Voice, especially Gretchen Young, Barbara Jones, and Marie Coolman, for believing in this project from its inception. To my editor at Hyperion, Sarah Landis, for your valuable comments and suggestions and for keeping the manuscript on track. To Dr. Julie Silver, at Harvard Health Publications, my deepest gratitude for your expertise and guidance with this project from the very start. You have become a true mentor. To my agent, Linda Konner, for making all the right connections and for your candid, spot-on advice. And to Jodie Gould, my writer, for making this adventure both enjoyable and fun. Thank you for making the science accessible and bringing shape to my vision. I am fortunate to be surrounded by such talented women!

To those working behind the scenes, including Rusty Shelton from Shelton Interactive, Robert (Duke) Bradley of CCTV, Debra Crosby of A Quest Actor's Studio, Dan Spinale and Jenna Hurley of Spinale and Co., journalist Cary Shuman, and photographer Patrick Lentz, as well as Diane Anderson and Lil Carter, Melissa Latham, and Mary Mahoney. I appreciate your support. To David Liscio, for your early contributions to the writing. And to Tim Maguire, for your time and generosity.

I am blessed with a loving family. To my parents, Richard and Patricia Burke, for giving me a secure foundation of love and the best education when money was tight. To my brothers, Rich, Mike, and Jude Burke, for your constant love and support—and especially to Rich, for bringing me to the anatomy lab during your first year of medical school and encouraging me to become a doctor.

To my sons, Eric and Stephen—you keep my brain young by sharing your love, your thoughts, and your life adventures. (Not to mention keeping me abreast of the latest technology!) Most of all, my deepest love and gratitude to my husband, Roger, my closest confidant, my personal medical editor, my athletic training partner, and my soul mate. Thank you for always encouraging me to step outside my comfort zone, for putting up with the countless Post-it notes that have adorned our home during the writing of this book, and most of all, Roger, thank you for your kindness and love.

—MP

I would like to thank Marie for helping me find new ways to open my eyes and my neural pathways. The more I see, the more I know.

My heartfelt thanks, as always, to my agent and friend Linda Konner, for her talent and tenacity.

And to Julie Silver, M.D., of Harvard Health Publications, for her creative guidance and support.

—JG

The references for the studies included in this book are listed on my Web site www.mariepasinski.com/book/references.